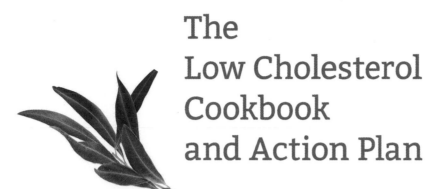

The
Low Cholesterol
Cookbook
and Action Plan

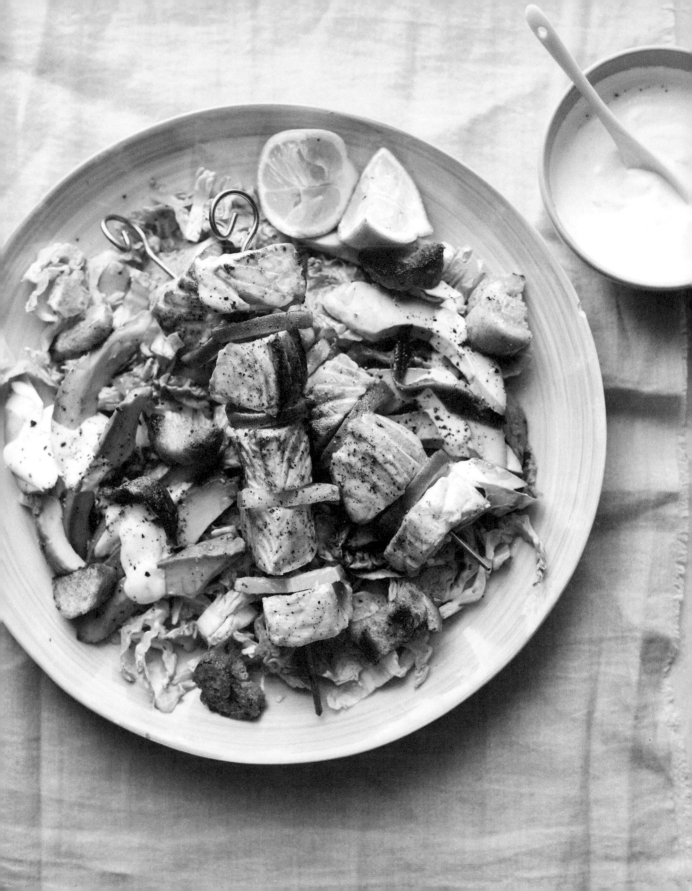

The
Low Cholesterol
Cookbook and Action Plan

4 Weeks to Cut Cholesterol and Improve Heart Health

KAREN L. SWANSON

with recipes by

JENNIFER KOSLO, PhD, RD, CSSD, ACE-CPT

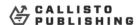
CALLISTO PUBLISHING

With love to Michael and Eric Lombardo, who were (mostly) enthusiastic as I experimented with lo-co recipes. And to my extraordinary writing group: Sari Bodi, Michaela MacColl, and Christine Pakkala.

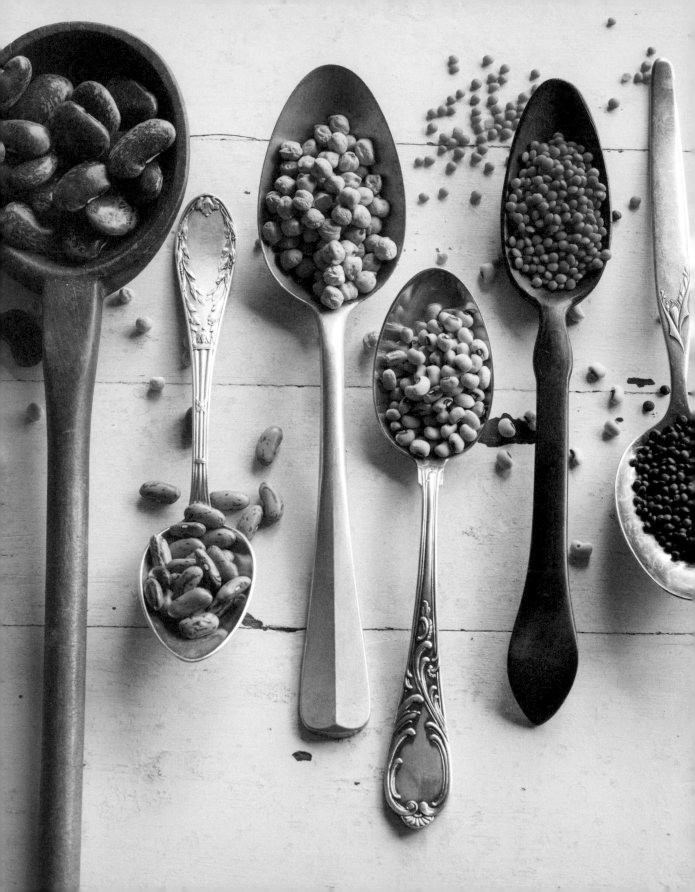

Contents

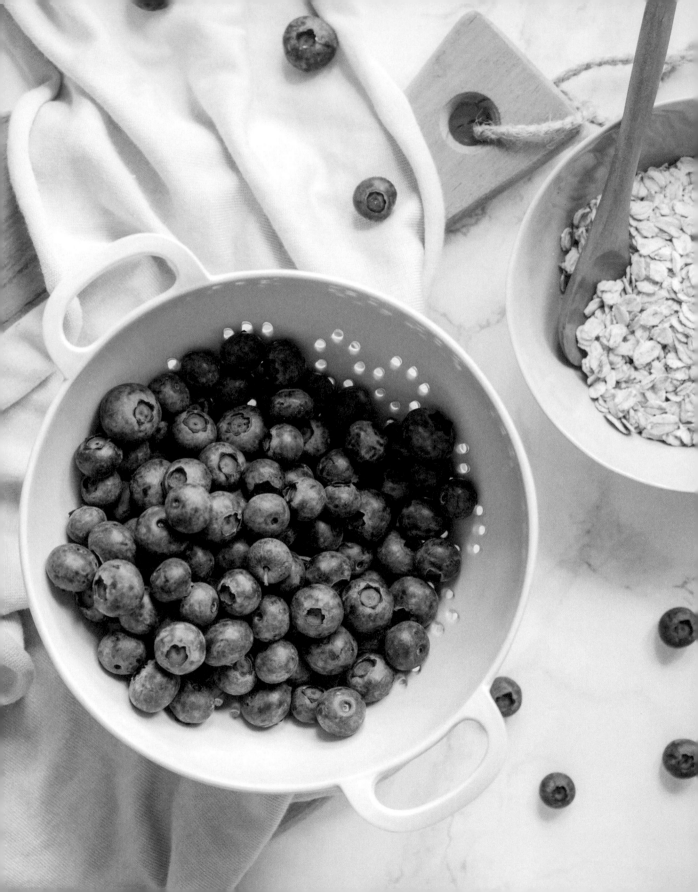

Introduction

There I was at my annual physical, waiting for my doctor to give me the usual news: "Your cholesterol is borderline high, but that runs in your family, right?" We'd then talk about diet and exercise and agree to keep an eye on it.

This time was different.

This time, she tapped her pen on her gray metal desk and frowned. She said that even though I was fit and healthy, my total cholesterol and LDL (bad) cholesterol levels had spiked past borderline. I was now at increased risk for heart disease and needed a cholesterol-lowering statin medication.

As nearly every adult in my family takes a statin, this should not have been a surprise to me—and, yet, I was stunned. When my doctor took out her prescription pad, I shook my head no—I knew that statins carry the potential for serious side effects. Instead I asked how to lower my cholesterol without medication.

She seemed concerned and reiterated the importance of treating high cholesterol early so plaque doesn't build in the arteries, which can cause a stroke or heart attack. In this moment I finally truly understood that my high cholesterol was a serious health risk and that I needed to take action to control it.

We agreed to try to lower my cholesterol naturally with diet and exercise if I promised to come back in six months for a new cholesterol test. After rummaging through her desk, she handed me a stapled copy of the DASH (Dietary Approaches to Stop Hypertension) diet. At my puzzled look, she explained it was for cholesterol, too.

I eagerly read the DASH diet, but it was woefully inadequate in guiding me toward a heart-healthy diet and exercise plan that was specific to lowering my cholesterol. So I started researching how to lower cholesterol on my own, and launched a blog to keep me committed to and accountable for exercising and eating more healthfully.

Changing habits is never easy, but after six months of slightly more exercise along with swapping red meat for lower-fat proteins and adding cholesterol-lowering foods, I was lifted out of the "needs a statin" group. Delighted, I kept at it. In seven years of living what I call a "lo-co" lifestyle, my cholesterol levels have stayed at an acceptable level.

It's a change that can benefit everyone—from those of us who need to lower cholesterol to those of us already managing heart disease. Put simply: Adopting a cholesterol-lowering approach to food and exercise reduces heart disease risk.

Making this shift is empowering. Finding new, healthier ways to cook that won't break the bank and don't taste or feel like a "diet" can actually be fun.

I'm excited to share with you how to transition to a lifestyle that can naturally lower your cholesterol. The goal of this book is not to drone on about cholesterol and its dangers. Rather, it's about creating a road map that includes achievable exercise goals and easy, delicious recipes. It's an action plan to jump-start your low-cholesterol lifestyle.

Let's get going!

PART ONE

....

GOING
LOW
CHOLESTEROL

Ready to go low cholesterol? Part 1 of this book describes how to lower cholesterol with food and exercise. First we'll cover the basics about cholesterol: what it is, how it's typically treated, and the role different foods and exercise play. Then we'll finish with a realistic food and exercise action plan designed to help naturally lower your cholesterol.

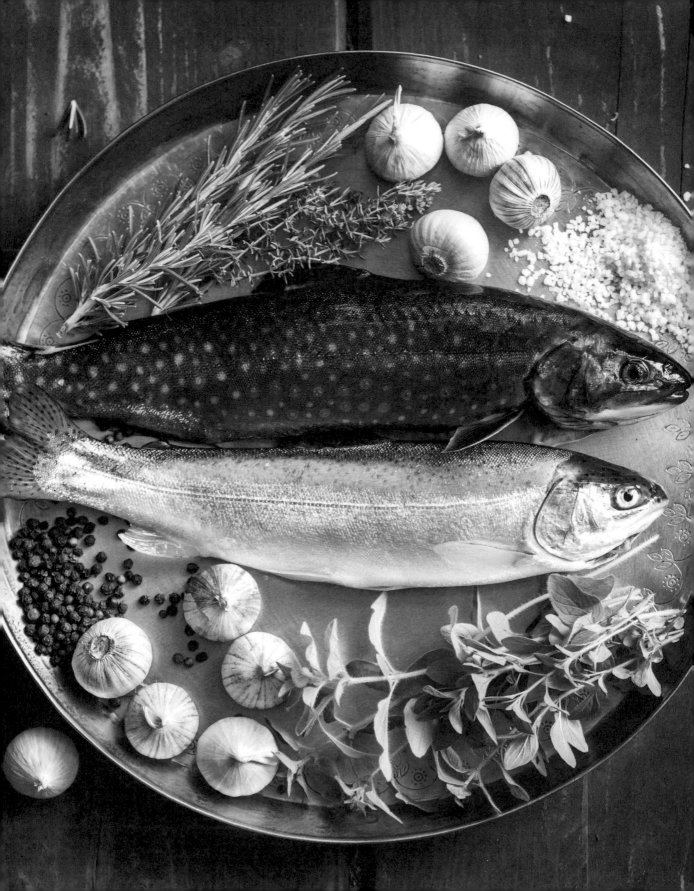

CHAPTER 1

Cutting Cholesterol

Like millions of Americans who want or need to lower their cholesterol, you may be wondering what exactly *cholesterol* is, why yours is high, and what you can do about it.

Cholesterol is a waxy, fatlike substance naturally produced by our bodies to help build cells. While it is not a fat, cholesterol is encased in lipids (fats) that enable it to travel through the bloodstream. Sources for more detailed information about cholesterol are included in the Resources section of this book (see page 193).

The problem is not that we have cholesterol—we naturally produce all we need. The issue is that a "typical" American diet contains too much saturated fat, which causes our livers to produce an overabundance of cholesterol, and a lack of exercise adds to that problem.

Your lifestyle—your food and exercise choices—is likely part of what caused your too-high cholesterol. The good news is that lifestyle changes can help you reverse that, and this book shows you how.

Understanding Cholesterol

High cholesterol is sneaky. It has no symptoms, but increases your risk of heart disease. When you don't have enough HDL (good) cholesterol, or you have too much LDL (bad) cholesterol, the excess cholesterol can accumulate and stick to the walls of your arteries as plaque.

When thick, hard plaque narrows the arteries and makes them less flexible (a dangerous condition known as *atherosclerosis* or "hardening of the arteries"), blood flow to the heart can become limited.

Your risk of developing high cholesterol depends on lifestyle choices you control, along with your genetics, medical conditions, age, gender, and ethnicity.

Risk Factors You CANNOT Control

Age. Your risk of developing high cholesterol increases with age.

Gender. Women have lower LDL (bad) cholesterol than men until around the age of menopause. In general, men have lower rates of HDL (good) cholesterol.

Ethnicity. While nearly one-third of all Americans have LDL cholesterol equal to or higher than 130 mg/dL,* non-Hispanic African American women have the highest percentage among women, and Mexican American men have the highest percentage among men.

Family history. Your risk is increased if high cholesterol runs in your family.

ABOUT CHOLESTEROL LEVELS

In a fasting cholesterol blood test, total cholesterol, LDL cholesterol, HDL cholesterol, and triglycerides are reported.

LDL cholesterol is often referred to as "bad" cholesterol because too much LDL cholesterol can cause plaque to build on the artery walls. The more LDL cholesterol in the blood, the greater the risk of heart disease.

HDL cholesterol is often called "good" cholesterol because it moves cholesterol to the liver, which eliminates it from the body. A higher HDL cholesterol level is desirable; a low count of HDL cholesterol increases the risk of heart disease.

Triglycerides are a type of fat found in blood, and high triglycerides increase heart disease risk, especially among women.

Diabetes. If you have diabetes, you have an increased risk of developing high cholesterol.

Risk Factors You CAN Control with Lifestyle Choices

Diet. A diet low in saturated fat, trans fat, salt, and sugar has been proven to lower cholesterol.

Exercise. All it takes is 40 minutes of moderate-to-vigorous aerobic exercise (brisk walking counts!) three to four times a week to lower both cholesterol and high blood pressure.

* Cholesterol is measured as milligrams (mg) per deciliter (dL) of blood.

How doctors treat high cholesterol has changed. In the past, statins were recommended if your cholesterol numbers were above target, but the latest medical guidelines focus on a 10-year risk of heart disease. Some doctors don't agree with this change, so there are some different opinions in the medical community on how to treat high cholesterol. But while medical controversy swirls, here's what's clear: Lowering cholesterol naturally with a (doctor-approved) heart-healthy food plan and frequent exercise is still a smart choice.

Smoking. Among other negative health effects, smoking actually lowers HDL (good) cholesterol.

Weight. Carrying excess weight puts you at risk for high cholesterol. Even a 10 percent weight loss can help lower your risk of high cholesterol.

Treating High Cholesterol

While everyone can help lower their own high cholesterol with heart-healthy lifestyle choices, if you have high cholesterol it is vital that you develop a plan with your doctor for reducing your heart disease risk.

One place to start—if you are over 40 and don't take a statin or have heart disease—is to check your 10-year heart disease risk using the Atherosclerotic Cardiovascular Disease (ASCVD) risk calculator (link provided in the Resources section, page 193), and discuss your results with your doctor.

If your risk of heart disease is high, your doctor may prescribe a cholesterol-lowering medication (a statin), and will likely advocate a

regular exercise plan and heart-healthy diet. If you smoke or are overweight, your doctor will work with you to reduce those risk factors, too.

Everyone can benefit from lowering their cholesterol with a change to a heart-healthy diet and regular exercise—but not everyone has taken that first step. So congratulations—you're already well on your way by picking up this book.

What Are Healthy Cholesterol Targets?

While a medical doctor's decision to treat high cholesterol with medication is now based on assessing a person's overall 10-year risk, rather than managing to a specific LDL target, the old methodology of assigning risk to certain cholesterol levels can still be useful. The following chart is from the National Institutes of Health. If your cholesterol results don't meet these levels, be sure to discuss any concerns with your doctor.

About Medication

Warning: While I can discuss medication, I am not a doctor and cannot make any recommendations. If your doctor has written you a prescription, it's important to follow that recommendation. Before making any substantial diet and exercise changes, discuss them with your doctor.

This book presents a drug-free approach to lowering cholesterol naturally. But only a doctor can judge whether your personal risk for heart disease is high enough to warrant medication. Here is an overview of the types of cholesterol-lowering medications your doctor might discuss with you.

Statins

The most common type of drug prescribed for lowering cholesterol is called a *statin*. Statins work by blocking the action of an enzyme in the liver needed to make cholesterol. Statins reduce LDL (bad) cholesterol and triglycerides.

Statins can have side effects—sometimes serious—which is why there are now questions about whether statins should be prescribed to those whose only heart disease risk is high cholesterol. Serious side effects, though rare, can include liver damage, type 2 diabetes, and muscle problems, which can range from myositis (essentially muscle inflammation) to rhabdomyolysis (extreme muscle inflammation and muscle damage.)

There are other cholesterol-lowering medications on the market. The chart on page 7, published by the Mayo Clinic, shows the types of medications, how they work, and their common side effects.

Who Needs a Statin?

Cholesterol-lowering statin medications are recommended for people age 40 to 75 years with one or more heart disease risk factors (high cholesterol, diabetes, high blood pressure, smoking) *and* a calculated 10 percent risk of a cardiac event in the next 10 years. Find a link to the ASCVD risk calculator in the Resources section (page 193).

HEALTHY CHOLESTEROL TARGETS

TOTAL CHOLESTEROL	ASSESSMENT
Less than 200 mg/dL	Desirable
200 to 239 mg/dL	Borderline high
240 mg/dL or higher	High

LDL (BAD) CHOLESTEROL	ASSESSMENT
Less than 100 mg/dL	Optimal
100 to 129 mg/dL	Near optimal/ above optimal
130 to 159 mg/dL	Borderline high
160 to 189 mg/dL	High
190 mg/dL or higher	Very high

HDL (GOOD) CHOLESTEROL	ASSESSMENT
Less than 40 mg/dL	A major risk factor for heart disease
40 to 59 mg/dL	The higher the better
60 mg/dL or higher	Considered protective against heart disease

TRIGLYCERIDES	ASSESSMENT
Less than 150 mg/dL	Normal
150 to 199 mg/dL	Borderline high: You may need treatment
200 mg/dL or higher	High: You may need treatment

DRUG CLASS AND NAMES	BENEFITS	POSSIBLE SIDE EFFECTS AND CAUTIONS
Statin Altoprev (lovastatin) Crestor (rosuvastatin) Lescol (fluvastatin) Lipitor (atorvastatin) Livalo (pitavastatin) Pravachol (pravastatin) Zocor (simvastatin)	Decreases LDL (bad cholesterol) and triglycerides; slightly increases HDL (good cholesterol)	Constipation, nausea, diarrhea, stomach pain, cramps, muscle soreness, pain, and weakness; possible interaction with grapefruit juice
Bile Acid Binding Resin Colestid (colestipol) Prevalite (cholestyramine) Welchol (colesevelam)	Decreases LDL (bad cholesterol)	Constipation, bloating, nausea, gas
Cholesterol Absorption Inhibitor Zetia (ezetimibe)	Decreases LDL (bad cholesterol); slightly increases triglycerides; slightly increases HDL (good cholesterol)	Stomach pain, fatigue, muscle soreness
Combination Cholesterol Absorption Inhibitor and Statin Vytorin (ezetimibe and simvastatin)	Decreases LDL (bad cholesterol) and triglycerides; increases HDL (good cholesterol)	Stomach pain, fatigue, gas, constipation, abdominal pain, cramps, muscle soreness, pain, and weakness; possible interaction with grapefruit juice
Fibrate Antara, Tricor, and others (fenofibrate) Lopid (gemfibrozil)	Decreases LDL (bad cholesterol) and triglycerides; increases HDL (good cholesterol)	Nausea, stomach pain
Niacin Niaspan, Niacor (prescription niacin)	Decreases LDL (bad cholesterol) and triglycerides; increases HDL (good cholesterol)	Facial and neck flushing, nausea, vomiting, diarrhea, gout, high blood sugar, peptic ulcers, itching
Combination Statin and Niacin Advicor (niacin and lovastatin)	Decreases LDL (bad cholesterol) and triglycerides; increases HDL (good cholesterol)	Facial and neck flushing, dizziness, heart palpitations, shortness of breath, sweating, chills; possible interaction with grapefruit juice
Omega-3 Fatty Acid Lovaza, Omtryg (prescription omega-3 fatty acid supplements) Vascepa (icosapent ethyl)	Decreases triglycerides; may increases HDL (good cholesterol)	Belching, fishy taste, indigestion
Combination Statin and Calcium Channel Blocker Caduet (atorvastatin and amlodipine)	Decreases LDL (bad cholesterol) and triglycerides; lowers blood pressure	Facial and neck flushing, dizziness, heart palpitations, muscle pain and weakness; possible interaction with grapefruit juice
Injectable Medication Praluent (alirocumab) Repatha (evolocumab)	Decreases LDL (bad cholesterol) in people with a genetic condition that causes very high LDL levels	Itching, swelling, pain or bruising at injection site, back pain, rash, hives, swelling of nasal passages, flu

Eating Your Way to Lower Cholesterol

Healthy eating to lower your cholesterol is not all about restriction, but, rather, moderation. Don't think of it so much as pining for red meat or the full-fat dairy foods you might be accustomed to, but as an opportunity to experience some new, delectable flavors.

There are four major food culprits that actually raise LDL (bad) cholesterol. Not to worry—it's not hard to replace these foods with heart-healthy choices, and there's a long list of healthy foods to add to your lo-co diet. Let's take a closer look.

What Not to Eat

The four key ingredients to **limit or avoid** are:

1. Saturated fats
2. Trans fats
3. Salt
4. Foods with added sugars

Our goal is to build a great tasting, easy-to-prepare, healthy eating approach that minimizes these foods.

First, a little more about fats: One of the most important things you can do to lower your cholesterol with a change in diet is to *minimize saturated fats and eliminate trans fats*. It's not the "dietary cholesterol" listed on the nutrition label that is most important; rather, it's whether the foods you eat contain these two "unhealthy" fats.

Why are saturated and trans fats so important to cut? Because these fats actually cause your liver to make even more cholesterol! In the article, "The Skinny on Fats," the American Heart Association (AHA) explains, "Knowing which fats raise LDL cholesterol and which ones don't is the first step in lowering your risk of heart disease and stroke. Your body naturally produces all the LDL cholesterol you need. Eating foods containing saturated fat and trans fat causes your body to produce even more, raising your blood cholesterol level."

SATURATED FATS

Avoiding saturated fats means staying away from three kinds of foods:

1. **Nonlean meat:** Saturated fat is largely found in animal products such as red meat (beef), lamb, pork, and poultry with skin.

2. **Dairy:** Saturated fat also lurks in dairy products, including butter, cream, cheeses, and foods made from whole or 2-percent milk.

3. **Oils:** Even plants can have saturated fats, especially the "tropical" oils (coconut oil, palm oil, and palm kernel oil), and cocoa butter.

TRANS FATS

Trans fats (also known as partially hydrogenated oils, or PHOs) are so unhealthy that in 2013 the US Food and Drug Administration (FDA) declared PHOs no longer "generally considered as safe." Trans fats are dangerous because they both raise LDL (bad) cholesterol and lower HDL (good) cholesterol.

Generally, trans fats are found in processed foods, such as baked goods and frozen foods, as well as fried fast foods. When cooking, you can avoid foods laden with trans fats by looking at the label: Since 2006 the FDA has required trans fats to be listed on Nutrition Facts labels. That said, products with less than 0.5 grams of trans fats per serving can state they contain "0 grams" trans fats, so it's also important to read the ingredient list: If "partially hydrogenated oils" is listed, avoid that food.

The FDA provides a list of foods that may contain partially hydrogenated oils:

- Coffee creamers

- Crackers, cookies, cakes, frozen pies, and other baked goods

- Ready-to-use frostings

- Refrigerated dough products, such as biscuits and cinnamon rolls

- Snack foods, such as buttered or flavored microwave popcorn, doughnuts

- Stick margarines

In "Prevention and Treatment of High Cholesterol," the AHA "recommends *limiting saturated fat to 5 to 6 percent of daily calories* and minimizing the amount of trans fat you eat." For someone eating 2,000 calories a day, that's about 11 to 13 grams of saturated fat. There is no set amount of trans fats—it's best not to have any.

SUGAR AND SALT

The other two foods to limit to lower cholesterol and heart disease risk are sugar and salt.

Most people eat far too much salt without even realizing it. The Centers for Disease Control and Prevention (CDC) report that "More than 75 percent of sodium Americans consume comes from processed and restaurant foods—not the salt shaker." This is vital, because too much salt

leads to high blood pressure, and having both high blood pressure and high cholesterol significantly increases heart disease risk. The AHA recommends the following amounts:

- No more than 2,300 milligrams (mg) a day for most adults

- Ideally, no more than 1,500 mg per day for most adults

Sugar has "long been cited for contributing to obesity, high blood pressure, and high cholesterol," according to the AHA's "Added Sugars Add to Your Risk of Dying from Heart Disease." The AHA recommends the following for sugar consumption:

- No more than 6 teaspoons of sugar, or 100 calories, a day for most women

- No more than 9 teaspoons, or 150 calories, a day for most men

What to Eat: Foods That Lower Cholesterol

A wide variety of foods actually help lower cholesterol. These foods tend to be low in saturated fat and high in fiber. The AHA and USDA recommend that a heart-healthy diet include:

- Lean meats and poultry, prepared using healthy fats and without the skin. The AHA advises to "select lean cuts of meat with minimal visible fat. Lean beef cuts include the round, chuck, sirloin, or loin. Lean pork cuts include the tenderloin or loin chop. Lean lamb cuts come from the leg, arm, and loin." The AHA also advises to buy "choice" or "select" grades rather than "prime," and select lean or extra-lean ground beef. Remove skin from chicken or turkey and trim all visible fat from meat before cooking. Limit processed meats such as salami, bacon, bologna, sausage, and hot dogs.

• Fish—especially fish high in omega-3 fatty acids—at least twice a week. It's delicious and easy to prepare. Fish delivers omega-3 fats, which lower LDL cholesterol and reduce triglycerides. According to the Mayo Clinic's "Cholesterol: Top Foods to Improve Your Numbers," the highest levels of omega-3 fatty acids are in mackerel, lake trout, herring, sardines, albacore tuna, salmon, and halibut.

• Foods containing "good" fats (monounsaturated and polyunsaturated fats) instead of foods high in "bad" fats (saturated and trans fats).

• Fat-free and/or low-fat dairy. Switch to low-fat or nonfat dairy and soy products.

• A variety of fiber-rich fruits and vegetables.

• Fiber-rich whole grains, rather than refined grains. At least half of all grains consumed should be whole grains. Healthier monounsaturated and/or polyunsaturated oils instead of oils high in saturated fat, which are solid at room temperature. Cook with liquid vegetable oils such as olive, canola, soybean, sunflower, and safflower oils.

Substituting these foods into your diet in place of the less healthy choices of the past can help lower your cholesterol naturally.

HEART-HEALTHY FOODS TO ADD TO YOUR DIET

Avocados: Like nuts, avocados are caloric—but they deliver monounsaturated fat, which can help lower LDL (bad) cholesterol. They are also rich in omega-3 fatty acids and are a fiber source.

Blueberries: These may support liver function, which helps wash out excess cholesterol.

Fiber-rich foods and fruits and vegetables: A diet high enough in fiber-rich foods is a diet that is going to lower cholesterol. Making fiber-rich foods, such as oatmeal and/or oat cereal, barley and other whole grains, beans, along with fruits and vegetables, a larger portion of your plate is a key step to naturally lowering cholesterol. The next section talks more about fiber, including its role in reducing cholesterol as well as listing specific fiber-rich foods.

Foods fortified with plant sterols and stanols: These block the body's ability to absorb cholesterol from food.

Nuts: Almonds, walnuts, hazelnuts, peanuts, pecans, and pistachios are rich in monounsaturated fat, fiber, and have vitamins and minerals that are heart-healthy. They also contain plant sterols. Eat about a handful (1.5 ounces, or 42.5 grams) a day, and make sure they aren't salted or coated with sugar. Use as a delicious, crunchy, heart-healthy snack or breakfast topping, but don't go overboard, as nuts have a lot of calories.

Seeds: Flaxseed and chia seeds are rich in omega-3 fatty acids.

Cholesterol by the Numbers

For those who like to go by the numbers, here are some targets to aim for.

A diet specific to lowering cholesterol doesn't strictly follow the USDA's *2015–2020 Dietary Guidelines for Americans*, which recommend 10 percent of calories per day come from saturated fats. A *heart-healthy diet,* according to the AHA, means *limiting saturated fats to 5 to 6 percent of daily calories* (based on 2,000 calories per day)— far less than the USDA guidelines.

So to lower cholesterol, our goal is to:

- Consume less than 5 to 6 percent of calories per day from saturated fats.

- Consume 25 grams of fiber per day (38 grams per day for men).

- Consume less than 10 percent of calories per day from added sugars.

- Consume less than 2,300 milligrams (mg) per day of sodium. Even better—especially for those at risk of high blood pressure—eat less than 1,500 mg per day. Why? Because limiting sodium is important for heart disease risk; both the AHA and the Mayo Clinic recommend a limit of 1,500 mg per day of sodium.

- Note that "dietary cholesterol" is not expressly stated in USDA guidelines any longer. A diet that meets these listed targets will, by default, limit dietary cholesterol consumption.

As saturated fat is so critical to reduce—and probably the area in which we need to change our habits the most—here's a guide published by the National Heart, Lung, and Blood Institute

If fast food is your only choice, choose grilled chicken—McDonald's Quarter Pounder with Cheese or Wendy's single cheeseburger each packs 13 grams of saturated fat, while a grilled chicken sandwich has just 1.5 grams. Add small fries, and the burger "meal" socks you with about 15 grams of saturated fat (more than the daily limit!), versus 3.5 grams for the chicken meal. See more tips for eating out in Appendix A, page 187.

that shows the maximum amount of saturated fat per day you need to target in order to reduce cholesterol:

IF YOU CONSUME:	EAT NO MORE THAN:
Calories per day	Saturated fat (amount = 6%)
1,200	8 grams
1,500	10 grams
1,800	12 grams
2,000	13 grams
2,500	17 grams

That means that those following the "typical" 2,000-calorie per day diet should aim for 13 grams of saturated fat for the entire day (for reference, there are 13 grams of fat in just one typical hamburger patty!).

The transition from eating foods high in saturated fats to foods low in saturated fats is a critical one. It may seem overwhelming at first, but it is doable. The recipes in this book give you the tips and tools to make this heart-healthy change easily and delectably.

Fight Cholesterol with Fiber

Dietary fiber is a critical component of a cholesterol-lowering diet. Fiber comprises both *soluble* and *insoluble* fiber. While both are important in digestive health, soluble fiber is the key to reducing cholesterol. Derived from plants, soluble fiber is a carbohydrate that cannot be broken down by your digestive system. It slows digestion and attaches to cholesterol as it moves through and out of your body. Five to 10 grams, or more, of *soluble* fiber each day decreases your total and LDL (bad) cholesterol levels.

In terms of *total* dietary fiber, the AHA specifies 25 grams of dietary fiber per day based on a 2,000-calorie diet.

To reach a goal of 25 grams of fiber per day, you'll want to ensure every meal and snack includes fiber. Here's one snapshot of the foods to eat in a day to achieve a 25-gram-per-day target; a broad list of fiber-rich foods is included at the end of this chapter.

In addition to other fruits, vegetables, and whole grains, these specific foods are high in cholesterol-lowering soluble fiber:

- **Apples, citrus fruits, grapes, and strawberries** have pectin, which is rich in soluble fiber.

- **Bananas** provide both soluble fiber and potassium.

- **Beans** are particularly rich in soluble fiber and are a good meat substitute because they are filling.

- **Blueberries, nuts, and seeds** are good sources of soluble fiber.

- **Oats** are high in soluble fiber, which binds to cholesterol and excretes it with bile acids.

HEART DISEASE RISK FACTORS

While high cholesterol is a significant risk factor for heart disease, there are other conditions that elevate risk. The more risk factors you have, the higher your chance of developing heart disease.

The National Heart, Lung, and Blood Institute lists the following conditions as heart disease risk factors. In addition, age (55 or older for women, 45 or older for men) increases your risk, so if you have one or more of these conditions, consult your doctor.

- Being overweight or obese

- Being physically inactive

- Diabetes or prediabetes

- Having a family history of early heart disease*

- Having a history of preeclampsia during pregnancy

- High blood cholesterol

- High blood pressure

- Smoking

- Unhealthy diet

* If your father or brother had a heart attack before age 55, or if your mother or sister had one before age 65, you are more likely to develop heart disease.

FIBER COMPONENT OF DAILY MEALS

	SERVING SIZE	DIETARY FIBER PER SERVING
TOTAL FOR DAY		25.9 grams
BREAKFAST		
Oatmeal	½ cup	4.0 grams
Topping: apple, almonds	½ apple, 0.5 ounce almonds	4.0 grams
Metamucil (Original Smooth, no sugar)	1 teaspoon	3.0 grams
LUNCH		
Sandwich on whole-wheat bread (Note: using peanut butter or fiber-rich avocado boosts fiber further.)	2 slices whole-wheat bread	3.8 grams
SNACK		
Herbed Chickpeas (page 78)	⅓ cup	4.4 grams
DINNER		
Sweet potato with skin on	½ medium	1.9 grams
Easy Roasted Asparagus, page 156	10 medium spears	3.0 grams
SNACK		
Air-popped popcorn	1.5 cups	1.8 grams

Eating oatmeal, or an oat cereal such as plain Cheerios, for breakfast delivers 1 to 2 grams of soluble fiber. Top it with any fiber-rich fruit, nut, and/or seed listed here for even more punch.

- **Peas, legumes, barley, quinoa, and other whole grains** deliver soluble fiber.

- **Psyllium fiber supplements,** taken daily, (Metamucil, Citrucel, FiberCon) deliver cholesterol-reducing fiber. Drink with cholesterol-lowering grapefruit juice* for even greater benefits. *__Warning:__ If you take *any* prescription medications—particularly blood pressure medications and some cholesterol-lowering medications—do not add grapefruit in any form to your diet without talking to your doctor. Grapefruit and grapefruit juice can affect the absorption rates of many medications.

Food Sources of Dietary Fiber

The table of foods high in dietary fiber per serving (page 14) is from the USDA's *2015–2020 Dietary Guidelines for Americans*. It's a handy tool to identify favorite foods you can eat to meet daily fiber goals.

DIETARY FIBER: FOOD SOURCES

Ranked by Amounts of Dietary Fiber and Energy per Standard Food Portions
and per 100 Grams of Foods

FOOD	STANDARD PORTION SIZE	CALORIES IN STANDARD PORTION*	DIETARY FIBER IN STANDARD PORTION (G)*	CALORIES PER 100 GRAMS*	DIETARY FIBER PER 100 GRAMS (G)*
High-Fiber Bran Ready-to-Eat Cereal	½ to ¾ cup	60–81	9.1–14.3	200–260	29.3–47.5
Navy Beans, Cooked	½ cup	127	9.6	140	10.5
Small White Beans, Cooked	½ cup	127	9.3	142	10.4
Yellow Beans, Cooked	½ cup	127	9.2	144	10.4
Shredded Wheat Ready-to-Eat Cereal (Various)	1–1¼ cup	155–220	5.0–9.0	321–373	9.6–15.0
Cranberry (Roman) Beans, Cooked	½ cup	120	8.9	136	10.0
Adzuki Beans, Cooked	½ cup	147	8.4	128	7.3
French Beans, Cooked	½ cup	114	8.3	129	9.4
Split Peas, Cooked	½ cup	114	8.1	116	8.3
Chickpeas, Canned	½ cup	176	8.1	139	6.4
Lentils, Cooked	½ cup	115	7.8	116	7.9

*US Department of Health and Human Services and US Department of Agriculture. *2015–2020 Dietary Guidelines for Americans*, 8th ed. December 2015. http://health.gov/dietaryguidelines/2015/guidelines/.

Making the Commitment

You have the tools—with your food and exercise choices—to help lower your cholesterol naturally. There will be bumps in the road; no change is ever easy. But you can do it.

In the beginning, it might take a bit more time in the kitchen and forethought than you are used to. You'll want to use a meal plan (see chapter 2) to ensure you have ingredients to make healthy choices all week. But it will soon become second nature for you to plan and make delicious, heart-healthy, cholesterol-lowering choices using the recipes in this book as a guide.

You might have food cravings or really miss your old style of eating—I know I did. Or you might find yourself flummoxed when looking at a restaurant menu. Remember, you don't need to be perfect; you just need to start choosing healthier foods. By making positive changes, little by little, you'll soon adjust to this healthier way of life.

As well, it's important not to get discouraged when you make some less-than-healthy choices. We all do it. Stay positive: There's always the next meal to make a different, healthier choice. Everything you do from this moment on that helps you embrace a cholesterol-lowering approach to food and exercise reduces your risk of heart disease.

Read on for how to make it happen for you.

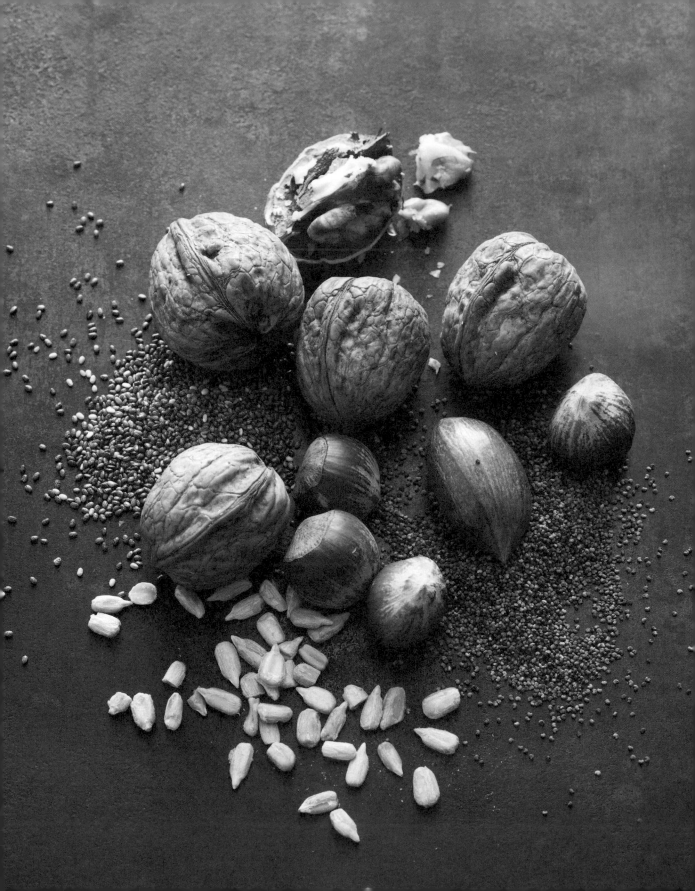

CHAPTER 2

5-Step Action Plan for Cutting Cholesterol

While naturally lowering your cholesterol requires a lifestyle change, I promise there will be no calorie counting, no hard-to-follow rules, and no crazy ingredients needed.

You will not have to adopt a radical exercise program. The exercise you need to lower cholesterol is a level that can be worked into a busy schedule. Even brisk walking counts!

I vow not to send you searching for expensive or hard-to-find ingredients, nor will you need chef-level skills to make these delicious heart-healthy recipes. I am a firm believer in making elegant, delicious food that is simple to prepare—using any and all cooking shortcuts. And while I can't guarantee that family members will like every recipe in this book, I am confident these are delectable dishes that most will enjoy and that do not taste like "diet" food. My philosophy is, "Don't tell them it's healthy; they'll just love the taste."

Let's launch your new low-cholesterol lifestyle, which I've broken down into five steps.

1. Clean the kitchen out.
2. Restock!
3. Prepare your kitchen.
4. Learn to meal plan.
5. Stay active.

Step 1:
Kitchen Clean-Out

For most of us, transitioning to a low-cholesterol eating style is a big shift, but it should feel manageable, not overwhelming. The best way to ditch old habits is by implementing small and simple changes, adopted at a rate that is comfortable for you.

Avoiding temptation is key: If you don't have food or ingredients that are high in saturated and trans fats in your pantry, refrigerator, or freezer, you can't eat them. As these are unhealthy for every person in your household, foods high in saturated fat and trans fats simply must go—and be replaced with heart-healthy choices.

The best way to start is to rid your kitchen of cholesterol-raising ingredients. These five types of foods have no place in your new heart-healthy cooking style and must be thrown out, given away, or donated:

High-fat dairy products. These include ice cream, full-fat milk, full-fat cheese and yogurt, sour cream, and the like.

Processed foods high in saturated fats and/or that contain trans fats or partially hydrogenated oils. These include sugary cereals, cookies, cakes, and crackers with hydrogenated oils, and bottled salad dressings, among other items.

Proteins high in saturated fat. These include high-fat cuts of red meat, and cured meats such as hot dogs, bacon, and sausage, as well as deli meats.

Refined grains. These include white rice and pasta.

Unhealthy oils. Butter,* any margarine that contains trans fats, all "tropical oils" (coconut and palm oils), all partially hydrogenated vegetable oils, and any oil or fat that is solid at room temperature.

Of course, it might not be possible to remove all these items. Perhaps you share your home with people who simply cannot live without some of these ingredients. That's okay; you can make it work by changing where these items are located. Store any heart-*un*healthy items in out-of-the-way places: Snacks could go in a basket or bin on a low shelf, refrigerated items could move to a back corner, not on the door. The idea is simple: If you do not see them, you will not be tempted to use them. And as a bonus, this strategy might help others in your household eat less of these heart-unhealthy foods!

Another obstacle might be your reaction to this list. If your thought upon reading it was, "But that's half of my kitchen!" that's totally understandable. In fact, you're right, because this is not a diet—it's a different approach to food. But not to worry, we're going to replace these heart-risky ingredients with heart-healthy items you'll love to cook with. And once your kitchen is stocked, you'll be ready to prepare food that will lower your cholesterol—and probably your weight, too!

---

* Butter might be the only exception, as a very small amount is sometimes desirable in recipes. While it would be best to remove butter from your household, it could potentially stay in your refrigerator if used sparingly and infrequently only in recipes, and you are not tempted to use it as a spread—ever.

GETTING SUPPORT FOR YOUR HEALTHY HABITS

While changing your approach to food is exciting, it can also be frustrating. Here are a few strategies to stay upbeat on your road to a low-cholesterol lifestyle:

Be kind to yourself. Try not to get too down on yourself if (when!) you make an unhealthy food choice: There's always the next meal to make a better choice. This is a journey.

Be patient and realistic with expectations. You've been eating your old way for years: It's not realistic to think you can change overnight. It will take time to develop new, healthier habits. But it can happen if you stick with it.

Change how you view the inevitable bumps in the road. Dr. Elizabeth Lombardo, author of *Better than Perfect:*

7 Strategies to Crush Your Inner Critic and Create a Life You Love, advises: "If you do slip up, apply my motto, 'It's not failure; it's data.' Use the data to understand your actions." Assess why you made that food choice: Were you feeling so hungry that you reached for a high-fat food? Or were you feeling stressed and needed a familiar comfort food? Understanding what caused a pitfall can help you remove it.

If your household or family members are not thrilled with your change in eating style, find ways to get them to collaborate with you. Here are some ideas:

- Alleviate whining by making everyone a part of meal planning. Instead of shouldering it all yourself, make it a household or family activity, where everyone gets to pick at least one dinner.

- Prepare just one dinner for all, but allow a self-made alternative (like cereal or a sandwich). You're not running a diner; you're in charge of a heart-healthy kitchen.

- If someone complains about missing an old favorite, challenge them to work with you on making a heart-healthy version of that recipe.

If you do get down or are feeling disappointed, remember it's okay to take things slowly. It's fine to try just one new, healthier food choice per day—that is progress you can build on. If you stay positive and view obstacles as challenges, your new healthier diet will simply become your new, healthier way of eating.

Step 2: Restock

Now that you've rid your kitchen of cholesterol-raising foods, it's time to restock with heart-healthy alternatives.

A cholesterol-lowering diet is rich in fruits and vegetables, so eating fresh, seasonal produce—when possible—is a great strategy. While many people prefer organic, locally grown, and free-range ingredients, it is certainly not necessary for a low-cholesterol cooking strategy. That said, avoiding pesticides is important; the Environmental Working Group's *Dirty Dozen* and *Clean Fifteen* lists are included in Appendix B (page 191) and help prioritize which foods are the most important to purchase as organic, and which are okay when you can't.

You can successfully create low-cholesterol meals regardless of whether you shop for fresh organic produce, or more affordable, more easily located ingredients. The most important thing is to control the amount of saturated fat and fiber in your meals, rather than defaulting to cholesterol-raising packaged, processed foods. Everyone, regardless of budget or taste preference, can cook to lower cholesterol.

The two main facts to check on Nutrition Facts labels as you restock your pantry are the *amount of fat* (saturated and trans fats) and the *amount of dietary fiber* in your restocking ingredients.

Saturated Fats

For most of us, the maximum amount of saturated fat we want to consume daily is 13 grams.

ON MARGARINE AND EGGS

People often have two questions about a cholesterol-lowering diet:

1. Is margarine healthier than butter?

2. Are eggs okay, or are they too high in dietary cholesterol?

Regarding butter versus margarine, the healthiest option is not to use a butter or margarine spread at all. But if a spread is absolutely necessary, a tub (not stick) margarine that contains no partially hydrogenated oils is a healthier choice. Tub margarines are made without partially hydrogenated oils, which are low in saturated fat and contain no trans fats. Check the label before you purchase any tub margarine spread.

Eggs—including yolks—are now considered part of a healthy diet, because the USDA has shifted its view on dietary cholesterol.

Eggs used to be considered unhealthy because they are high in dietary cholesterol (one large egg contains about 210 mg of dietary cholesterol and the daily limit was 300 mg). But the USDA now recommends eggs as a healthy protein. It is now believed that consuming saturated fat, not dietary cholesterol, is the culprit in raising cholesterol and heart disease risk.

To do that, look for lean proteins and ingredients designated as "low in saturated fat." The US FDA classifies food as low in saturated fat if it contains *1 gram or less per serving*.

Dietary Fiber

To reach a target of 25 grams of dietary fiber per day, stock up on oats, beans, and grains, which are very high in dietary fiber, along with fresh fruits and vegetables. Chapter 1 includes the USDA Dietary Guidelines list of foods high in dietary fiber per serving (page 14); it is a great reference as you restock your pantry.

The following are some general pantry guidelines for ingredients that are great to have on hand. Note that the meal plans contain separate pantry lists, and some recipes contain "Budget Saver" tips—which are also time-savers—that use frozen, dried, or canned ingredients.

Restock with Heart-Healthy Staples

When your kitchen is stocked with low-fat, fiber-rich ingredients, it's easier to prepare heart-healthy meals. The following broad list serves as a guideline. You don't need every item:

The AHA's Heart-Check label can help you easily identify heart-healthy foods. If you see this mark [insert AHA icon] on an ingredient, food, or menu item, you'll know that food has limited saturated fat, trans fat, sodium, and sugar. Specifically, foods with this label contain 1 gram or less of saturated fat per serving, and less than 0.5 gram of trans fats.

Choose what looks appealing, at quantities that fit how often you like to grocery shop.

PANTRY BASICS

Barley, hulled

Beans, a wide variety of dried and canned beans, no-salt-added, especially black beans, cannellini beans, chickpeas, kidney beans, and navy beans

Breads, whole-wheat

Broth, canned, chicken, low-sodium

Cereals, wheat bran and oat-based

Chilies, diced, canned

Dried peas and lentils

Herbs and spices, fresh and dried, a variety

Mustard, whole-grain and Dijon, preferably low-salt

Nuts, raw, unsalted, a variety

Oatmeal, old-fashioned rolled oats and/or steel-cut oats

Pasta, whole-grain

Peanut butter, natural (made with just peanuts and a bit of salt)

Popping corn

Psyllium fiber supplement

Quinoa, prewashed makes preparation much easier

Rice, brown

Seeds, chia, flax, pumpkin, and sunflower

Tomato sauce, no-salt-added, canned

Tomatoes, diced, no-salt-added, canned

Tomatoes, sun-dried, dry-packed

Vinegars, flavored, a variety

VEGETABLES

Canned, such as baby peas, carrots, mushrooms, and no-salt-added diced tomatoes

Frozen, such as broccoli, cauliflower, mixed, spinach, and string beans

Garlic

Greens, fresh, leafy and fresh vegetables of every color

Onions

Potatoes, skin-on

Ready-to-use fresh vegetables: already-cubed butternut squash, pre-diced onion, and spiralized zucchini

Shallots

Sweet potatoes, skin-on

PROTEINS

Beef, which should be avoided, but if essential choose "extra lean"

Chicken and turkey, skinless, dark or white meat, fresh or frozen; white meat is preferable, but any skinless chicken or turkey is a better choice than red meat

Eggs

Legumes (beans and peas)

Pork, lean cuts such as loin chops or tenderloin

Shellfish, such as clams, mussels, scallops, shrimp, and squid, fresh or frozen

Tuna, low-sodium, packed in water or a vacuum-sealed pouch, canned

FRUIT

Apples, skin-on

Avocados

Bananas

Berries, fresh and frozen

Citrus

Dates

Guava

Pears, skin-on

DAIRY

Cheese, fat-free or low-fat shredded (check sodium levels); fat-free or low-fat feta; Parmesan, fresh or freshly grated (with no preservatives)

Milk, dairy, fat-free (skim) or low-fat

Milk, nut, almond or cashew

Milk, soy

Sour cream, fat-free or low-fat

Yogurt, fat-free or low-fat traditional or Greek-style

FATS AND OILS

Canola oil

Liquid or soft margarine, made with vegetable oil. The first ingredient must be unsaturated liquid vegetable oil (not hydrogenated or partially hydrogenated oil)

Olive oil

Your choice of other unsaturated oils in addition to olive and canola, including corn, safflower, sesame, soybean, and sunflower

Step 3: Prepare Your Kitchen

No equipment beyond the usual pots and pans, knives, cutting boards, whisks, and spatulas is necessary to start your cholesterol-lowering cooking journey. But since you'll likely be spending more time in the kitchen than before, it can be a big help to have kitchen tools that make it easier to get your cooking done.

Kitchen Essentials

To support your low-cholesterol cooking style, here are a few recommended essential kitchen items.

Nonstick Skillet(s) with Lid(s). Limiting your use of oils when cooking works best with nonstick pans. There are many options beyond the original scratch-prone Teflon, including light-weight cast-iron skillets covered in durable, nonstick porcelain. You will likely want at least two skillets—one small or medium size and one large enough to prepare food for several people, or batch cook for the week. Great nonstick skillets do not have to cost a lot; there are many reputable online reviews to help determine your best option.

Rimmed Baking Sheets. Roasting a big batch of vegetables is a great way to ensure a supply of healthy, high-fiber ingredients for use in multiple meals. Tossing cut-up vegetables with a bit of olive oil and salt and roasting on a rimmed baking sheet lined with nonstick aluminum foil is a fast, no-cleanup method to prepare just about any vegetable. Your baking sheets do not need to be fancy, but they do need a rim so your vegetables will not fly off when you take them out of the oven! Also, make sure you can fit two sheets side by side in your oven—I learned the hard way that some sheets are too long to fit in my oven!

Pots. You will need a basic assortment of pots with lids to make pasta, rice, and grains, and to cook or heat a variety of foods.

Measuring, Mixing, and Storage Containers. While you do not need a kitchen scale or special measuring tools, you will need basic measuring cups and spoons, along with assorted mixing bowls. Airtight containers for storing the healthy ingredients you batch cook, and for leftovers, are also essential.

Knives and Cutting Boards. It is easier and safer to prepare foods when you have a sharp knife and a clean cutting board. Your knives do not need to be expensive; they just need to be sharp and able to hold an edge. At minimum, you will want a chef's knife and a paring knife. With cutting boards, wood is easiest on knives; bamboo cutting boards are great for fruits and vegetables. Dedicating a plastic cutting board to use with raw meats is a good idea, as these can be sanitized in the dishwasher.

Blender or Food Processor. To make smoothies, purée soups, slice onions without crying, or pulverize nuts to make homemade nut butters, nothing beats a food processor. A less-expensive option for making smoothies and soups is a high-powered blender.

Nonstick Aluminum Foil and Parchment Paper. When you do not have, or want to spend, a lot of time for cleanup, a sheet of nonstick aluminum foil or parchment paper to line a roasting pan or a baking sheet is indispensable.

Nice to Have

While the following items are not essential, they can make your low-cholesterol cooking a lot more enjoyable.

Olive Oil Mister. Why pay for cooking spray made from ingredients not listed on the can, when you can create your own for free, using heart-healthy olive oil? For about $10, you can get an olive oil mister you fill with your own olive oil. Every time you want to slick a pan or your ingredients with olive oil, just pump the sprayer to prime it, then mist freely. It is one of my favorite tools, as it makes it nearly impossible to douse a pan or ingredients with too much oil.

Mandoline. A mandoline helps you slice vegetables very thinly, without the bother or expense of a food processor. While traditional mandolines have multiple pieces and can be expensive, one-piece, handheld mandolines are available for less than $25. Mandoline blades are extremely sharp—be extra careful when using, cleaning, and storing them.

Rice Cooker. Rice cookers cook far more than just rice! You can make quinoa, oatmeal, and many other grains in rice cookers. Plus, there is no need to worry about timing as they switch to the Keep Warm setting once done. Some even have vegetables steamers to cook fresh vegetables simultaneously. Rice cookers come in small, medium, and large sizes, at affordable prices.

Slow Cooker. To easily make high-fiber, steel-cut oatmeal, or come home to an already-cooked, heart-healthy meal, a slow cooker is a fantastic tool. Choose one with a removable insert that can go into the dishwasher for the most flexibility.

Yogurt Maker. Avoid sugar-laden, store-bought yogurt by making your own. While homemade yogurt is easy to make and requires no special tools, it can be tricky to time, as you must refrigerate it after 12 hours. While expensive, a yogurt maker that automatically switches to refrigeration eliminates the timing obstacle.

Step 4:
Learn to Meal Plan

Meal planning is key, as it helps ensure you have all you need to successfully cook a week's worth of the cholesterol-lowering, heart-healthy meals you deserve. It also saves time and money, and fends off the dreaded question: "What's for dinner?"

Here are five easy steps to meal planning:

1. **Match your calendar commitments with cooking plans.** Decide which days of the upcoming week you'll have time to cook (30 to 45 minutes, not hours!) versus which days are short on time and are better for slow cooker meals, leftovers, or a meal that uses batch cooked or canned ingredients. Starting with a realistic plan sets you up for success.

2. **Plan meals that fit your cooking plans.** Slot into each weekday the type of meal you have time to prepare. Use the following grid as a guide to match your available time with a recipe type; this can significantly reduce the stress of getting dinner on the table—and make cooking more fun—because you'll have enough time to prepare a great meal.

3. **Choose recipes that fit.** Choose recipes that fit your cooking plans and available time, and review the plan to make sure there is a variety of proteins and grains so your week is full of delicious, varied foods. Bonus tip: Choosing recipes with shared ingredients saves time and money.

Don't forget about breakfast, lunch, and snack planning. Have a hankering for leftovers for lunch? Choose recipes that travel well. And always consider what you can batch cook to yield healthy, nutritious meal options all week long.

All the recipes in this book are low in saturated fat, so you're covered there. But does your meal plan deliver enough daily fiber? Take a look at both breakfast and snacks, and make sure those help you reach the target of 25 grams of daily fiber.

4. **Make an ingredient list and a shopping list.** Once you have selected your recipes for the week, make a master ingredient list that includes all the ingredients from every recipe. Check it against what's already stocked in your refrigerator, freezer, or pantry to create a shopping list.

30 MINUTES TO 1 HOUR	30 MINUTES TO 1 HOUR	15 TO 20 MINUTES	10 MINUTES	NO TIME
Make a recipe just for tonight	Make a recipe with leftovers for tomorrow	Assemble a dinner using leftovers or precooked ingredients	Slow cooker dinner	Dine out or takeout from restaurant with heart-healthy choices

If you organize your list by grocery category, your shopping trip will be more efficient. I use an app called AnyList that not only organizes items by category (you cross off items with a simple tap), it also enables sharing—so anyone in the household can add a grocery item at any time.

5. **Batch cook and prep!** Once you've selected your recipes for the week and have all your food gathered, it's time to prep and cook. It's far easier to stick with a heart-healthy meal plan when you prep for the week by cooking a big batch of grains, roasting lots of vegetables, and washing and storing fresh fruit in single-serve portions.

To kick off your cholesterol-lowering meal planning, the next chapter includes a four-week meal plan with a shopping list for each week. You can customize and mix and match, but this should help you jump right into heart-healthy meal planning.

Step 5: Stay Active

Besides helping lower cholesterol, daily exercise—even just brisk walking—will help you sleep better and lift your mood, and can also result in weight loss.

For general health, the AHA recommends that everyone gets 150 minutes per week of moderate exercise. That's 30 minutes a day, five days a week—and walking counts! So, at minimum, we all need to walk at least 30 minutes daily.

To lower cholesterol and blood pressure, you need to do a little bit more (but it's still not a lot!).

For lowering cholesterol, the AHA recommends 40 minutes of moderate-to-vigorous intensity aerobic exercise, three to four times a week.

If 40 minutes at once sounds like a lot— or you don't have a 40-minute block in your day—you can still easily get to this level of cholesterol-lowering exercise by breaking it up into two or three segments of 10 to 20 minutes per day.

So what's moderate-to-vigorous exercise? The CDC defines it in the table on page 28.

Do Cardio

When you're breathing hard and your heart rate elevates, you know you're getting cardiovascular exercise—an important component in preventing heart disease and stroke. If you play tennis, swim laps, or take a spin class, you're getting cardio. Do these three to four times a week, and you're getting the cholesterol-lowering exercise you need.

MyFitnessPal is a surprisingly easy-to-use app that can help you quickly make better choices at fast-food restaurants, and keep track of both your exercise and how much fiber and saturated fat you consume daily. Because this app has such a large food database, it is shockingly easy and quick to record every meal and snack. Use it to get a real-time sense of your successes and areas needing improvement. You can even enter your own recipes and it will calculate their nutritional value. It's one of my absolute favorite tools.

There are many other no-cost, nonsporty, no-gym ways to boost cardiovascular fitness.

- Go for a brisk walk or a slow jog for 40 minutes. Or take two 20-minute brisk walks or slow jogs. Or take three or four breaks from work and get some brisk walking in that way.

- Take the stairs—always, wherever you are, all day. At home, you can do sets of 10-minute climbs, up and down your own steps.

- Bike to work.

- Jump rope and do jumping jacks.

- Take 10-minute dance breaks with your kids—or by yourself.

Build Strength

It's always important to talk with your doctor before beginning any kind of exercise program. The AHA recommends strength training at least twice per week. The concept behind strength training is to push and pull weight. It can be your own bodyweight, free weights, resistance bands, or even objects from your home, such as cans of soup.

Here are a few strength-training exercises you can do at home. Do them in groups of 10, resting between sets. If you're not sure about form, there are many online resources.

- Biceps curls
- Lunges
- Push-ups
- Sit-ups

Get Loose

As we age, our muscles stiffen, which can lead to injury. Stretching helps by elongating the muscles in our bodies. The Mayo Clinic offers a free online guide to basic stretches, with visuals. It's important to warm up for 5 to 10 minutes before any stretching—even better is to stretch after exercising, when your muscles are warm. Stretch slowly, remembering to breathe, and hold each stretch for 10 to 30 seconds without bouncing. Switch sides and repeat. Try these:

Hamstring Stretch. The hamstring—the large muscle that runs from your knee to your hip on the back of the thigh—often gets tight, and that can lead to back pain. Here is one way to stretch your hamstrings: Sitting in a chair, with another chair facing you about one leg-length away, extend your left leg out in front of you, placing your left heel on the chair opposite. Lean forward until you feel the stretch in the back of your thigh. Do not bounce. If it hurts, you are stretching too far. Repeat with the right leg. As your flexibility improves, lean farther forward on each stretch.

Hip Flexor Stretch. Your hip flexors are located on your upper thighs, just below your hipbones. As with hamstrings, tight hip flexors can cause back pain. To stretch your hip flexors: Kneel with your right knee on a towel and plant your left foot flat on the floor, directly under your bent left knee. Place your left hand on your left thigh for stability. Keeping your back straight and abdominal muscles tight, lean forward, shifting your body weight onto your front leg: You'll feel a stretch in your right thigh. (You can place your

SUGGESTED MODERATE AND VIGOROUS ACTIVITIES

MODERATE ACTIVITY	VIGOROUS ACTIVITY
Walking at a 3- to 4.5-mile-per-hour pace (That's a 20- to 13-minute-per-mile pace)	Walking or jogging at a 5-mile-per-hour or faster pace (That's a 12-minute-per-mile pace or faster)
Biking on level terrain at 5 to 9 miles per hour	Biking on hills and/or at 10 miles per hour or faster
Stationary bicycling with moderate effort	Stationary bicycling with high effort (spin class)
Aerobics or water aerobics	Step aerobics or water jogging
Light calisthenics	Vigorous calisthenics
Yoga	Karate, judo, tae kwon do
Hiking	Mountain climbing
Stair climber or rowing machine with light effort	Stair climber or rowing machine with high effort
Tennis: doubles	Tennis: singles
Swimming: recreational	Swimming: laps
Light gardening or yard work	Gardening or yard work with heavy digging
General housework	Heavy housework

Centers for Disease Control and Prevention. "General Physical Activities Defined by Level of Intensity." www.cdc.gov/nccdphp/dnpa/physical/pdf/pa_intensity_table_2_1.pdf

right hand on your right hip to avoid bending at the waist). Hold for about 30 seconds. Switch legs and repeat.

Knee to Chest Stretch.* This stretches your lower back. On a floor or other hard surface, lie on your back with your heels flat on the floor and toes pointing up. Gently pull one knee to your chest until you feel a slight stretch in your lower back, keeping the opposite leg relaxed and straight. (It is okay to have the knee bent on the leg you are not holding.) Hold for about

30 seconds. Switch legs and repeat. ***Warning:** *This stretch should not be done if you have osteoporosis or back issues, without consulting your physician.*

Shoulder Stretch. Tight shoulders can cause rotator cuff problems: Stretch your shoulders to keep them flexible. Standing tall, bring your left arm across your chest and hold it with your right forearm, either above or below the elbow. Hold for about 30 seconds. Switch arms and repeat.

Improve Flexibility

Yoga is a fantastic way to improve flexibility and relieve stress. While some people love yoga classes, others don't have the time or money to go to a studio, or might feel uncomfortable in public. Don't let any of those roadblocks get in your way; you can find great, free yoga programs for beginners (and other levels) online. Search for one that's right for you.

Maintaining Motivation

The key to successfully changing to a cholesterol-lowering, heart-healthy lifestyle is to view all this as an exciting journey. Be patient with yourself and don't expect perfection. Work your way into an exercise program that you enjoy.

As for diet, expect ups and downs: Know that not every day—or even every meal—will be perfect. Remember to be kind to yourself as you embark on this change to a new way of life. Have some fun with it. Keep track of your daily steps or general exercise progress using apps, smart watches, spreadsheets, pen and paper—whatever works to motivate you.

Be sure to celebrate your cooking successes. Award smiley-face emojis or stars to the heart-healthy recipes you love. Tweak them to reflect your personal tastes to bring this cookbook to life and make it your own.

Congratulations on taking the first step to a cholesterol-lowering, heart-healthy lifestyle. Here's wishing you much enjoyment and success on your heart-healthy journey.

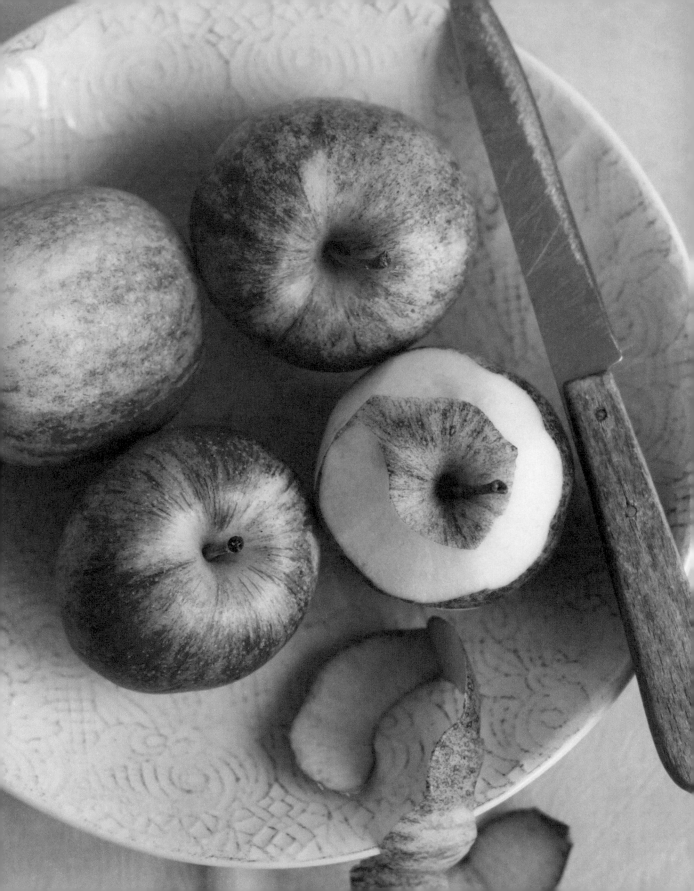

CHAPTER 3

The Plan

This section details a suggested four-week meal plan and suggested physical activity plan to help you get started on lowering your cholesterol. The meal plans and shopping lists are for one person, so if you are cooking for others, remember to double or triple the quantities as necessary.

The recipes used in the meal plans serve from one to four people, which is great if you are cooking just for yourself—you can cook once and have leftovers for additional meals—or if you are a cholesterol-minded couple, or if you are caring for an individual who is battling health issues. The weekly shopping lists are designed to be budget-friendly and minimize waste.

The midmorning and midafternoon snacks are suggestions; everyone has different calorie needs depending on their gender, age, and level of physical activity. Aim to include a balance of nutrients and modify the portions to fit your hunger level and energy needs. Afternoon snacks are larger, to provide energy for the afternoon, and they include lean protein, healthy fats, and carbohydrates to fuel your activity. Use the food group suggestions to mix and match and come up with your own healthy combinations.

As a reminder, at minimum, for general health the AHA recommends 150 minutes per week of moderate exercise. That's 30 minutes a day, five days a week—and brisk walking counts!

To lower cholesterol and blood pressure, the AHA recommends 40 minutes of moderate-to-vigorous intensity aerobic exercise, three to four times a week. If you don't have a 40-minute block in your day, get your minutes in by breaking it up into two or three segments of 10 to 20 minutes each.

To review moderate-to-vigorous exercise options, see page 28.

Always talk with your doctor before beginning any kind of exercise program. And if you've been sedentary, talk with your doctor about the best way to start exercising and how to work your way up to more vigorous exercise.

By sticking with a healthy eating and physical activity plan, you should soon see positive changes in your blood cholesterol readings.

SERVING SIZE GUIDE

Fruits and Vegetables:

1 cup fresh fruits and vegetables or 100% fruit juice = 1 cup serving; ½ cup dried fruit = 1 cup serving; 1 cup cooked or raw = 1 cup serving; 2 cups leafy greens = 1 cup serving

Proteins, including meats, seafood, poultry, beans and peas, eggs, soy products, and nuts and seeds:

Meat is measured in ounces; 1 egg = 1 ounce; ½ ounce of nuts or seeds = 1-ounce serving

Grains:

1 slice bread; 1 cup dry cereal; ½ cup cooked grains or pasta = 1-ounce serving

Dairy:

1 cup milk or yogurt = 1 serving; cheese differs on how it was processed, so for natural cheese, 1½ ounces = 1 serving and for processed cheese, 2 ounces = 1 serving

Oils:

Measured in teaspoons not ounces, and 1 tablespoon vegetable oil, 1 ounce dry nuts, or half a medium avocado = 1 tablespoon of oil

The USDA recommends the following servings per day for a 2,000-calorie diet:

2 cups fruit

2½ cups vegetables

6 ounces grains

5½ ounces protein

3 cups dairy

Oil and discretionary calories, as well as exact serving-size requirements, are based on each individual person's age, gender, and activity level. Go to the USDA's ChooseMyPlate.gov to enter your personal information and determine the specific amount of each food group you needed daily.

	BREAKFAST	SNACK	LUNCH	SNACK	PHYSICAL ACTIVITY	DINNER
SUNDAY	Creamy Oat Bran with Apricots, page 62 (makes 2 servings)	1 serving fruit or vegetable (e.g., 1 apple or 1 cup baby carrots)	4 ounces grilled skinless chicken breast, 1 cup steamed vegetables, 1 slice whole-grain bread	1 hardboiled egg with 1 cup baby carrots	Walk briskly for 30 minutes	Steamed Rosemary Trout in Parchment with Spinach, page 118 (makes 4 servings)
MONDAY	Leftover Creamy Oat Bran with Apricots, page 62	1 serving fruit or vegetable (e.g., 1 apple or 1 cup baby carrots)	Leftover Steamed Rosemary Trout in Parchment with Spinach, page 118	1 cup low-fat plain Greek yogurt	Walk briskly for 30 minutes	Slow Cooker White Beans and Barley, page 82 (makes 4 servings, freeze 1)
TUESDAY	Bowl of oat cereal with low-fat milk, 6 ounces Greek yogurt, fresh berries	1 serving fruit or vegetable (e.g., 1 apple or 1 cup baby carrots)	Leftover Slow Cooker White Beans and Barley, page 82	1 ounce unsalted nuts with 1 medium piece of fruit	Walk briskly for 30 minutes	Oatmeal-Crusted Chicken Tenders, page 103 (makes 4 servings)
WEDNESDAY	Pear Pistachio Overnight Oats, page 60 (makes 2 servings)	1 serving fruit or vegetable (e.g., 1 apple or 1 cup baby carrots)	Leftover Oatmeal-Crusted Chicken Tenders, page 103, over 2 cups mixed baby greens with avocado slices	½ cup low-fat cottage cheese with 1 medium piece of fruit	Walk briskly for 30 minutes	Leftover Steamed Rosemary Trout in Parchment with Spinach, page 118
THURSDAY	Cranberry-Orange Muffin in a Mug, page 55 (1 serving)	1 serving fruit or vegetable (e.g., 1 apple or 1 cup baby carrots)	Leftover Steamed Rosemary Trout in Parchment with Spinach, page 118	1 cup low-fat plain Greek yogurt	Walk briskly for 30 minutes	4 ounces grilled skinless chicken breast, 1 cup steamed vegetables, ½ cup brown rice, green salad
FRIDAY	Leftover Pear Pistachio Overnight Oats, page 60	1 serving fruit or vegetable (e.g., 1 apple or 1 cup baby carrots)	Leftover Oatmeal-Crusted Chicken Tenders, page 103, over 2 cups mixed baby greens with avocado slices	1 ounce unsalted nuts with 1 medium piece of fruit	Walk briskly for 30 minutes	Leftover Slow Cooker White Beans and Barley, page 82
SATURDAY	Bowl of oat cereal with low-fat milk, 6 ounces Greek yogurt, fresh berries	1 serving fruit or vegetable (e.g., 1 apple or 1 cup baby carrots)	Leftover Oatmeal-Crusted Chicken Tenders, page 103, over 2 cups mixed baby greens with avocado slices	1 low-fat string cheese with 1 medium piece of fruit	Walk briskly for 30 minutes	4 ounces grilled pork tenderloin, 1 cup steamed vegetables, baked sweet potato, green salad

Suggested Menu and Activity. Meals in blue are recipes from this book. Use the other meal suggestions as a guide, or swap them for recipes in this book. The physical activity can be done when it suits your schedule the best, but aim to be active each day for at least 30 minutes.

Check your pantry and refrigerator for:

Almonds, raw, unsalted
Baby greens, mixed
Fresh fruit and berries
Garlic
Milk, nonfat or low-fat,
    dairy or soy

Nonstick cooking spray
Oats, old-fashioned rolled
Olive oil
Onions
Peanut butter or other nut or
    seed butter, unsalted

Pepper
Salt
Sweetener of choice, such
    as stevia, pure maple
    syrup, honey
Vinegar of choice

Shop for:

FRESH PRODUCE: SNACKS
Fresh fruit and fresh vege-
    tables: a combination of
    12 servings (you can also
    use canned fruit in light
    syrup or unsweetened dried
    fruit), including apples and
    baby carrots

FRESH PRODUCE: MEALS
Apricots, 4 (or dried,
    unsweetened)
Avocados, 2
Berries, 1 pint container
Carrots, 2 medium
Cranberries, ¼ cup
Greens, salad, mixed 10 cups
Mushrooms, portobello, 4
Orange, navel, 1
Onion, 1 medium
Pears, 2 medium
Rosemary, 1 small bunch
Shallots, 4
Spinach, baby, 2 cups
    (about 5 ounces)
Sweet potato, 1 medium
Thyme, 1 small bunch

FROZEN PRODUCE
Mixed vegetables,
    1 (16-ounce) package
Spinach, 1 (10-ounce) package

GRAINS
Barley, hulled, 1 cup
Bread, whole-grain, 1 loaf
Rice, brown, ½ cup

DAIRY
Cottage cheese, low-fat,
    1 small (8-ounce) container
Milk, low-fat, soy or dairy,
    4 cups
Parmesan cheese, freshly
    grated, ½ cup
String cheese, low-fat,
    1 string cheese
Yogurt, low-fat Greek,
    4½ cups
Yogurt, nonfat, vanilla,
    2 tablespoons

EGGS
2 large

GROCERY ITEMS
Baking powder, ½ teaspoon
Beans, white, 1 (15-ounce) can

Broth, vegetable, low-sodium,
    32 ounces
Cereal, oat bran, 1 box
Cinnamon, ground,
    ¼ teaspoon
Flour, oat, 1 tablespoon
Nut butter of choice, unsalted,
    1 tablespoon
Nut of choice, raw, unsalted,
    2 ounces
Oats, old-fashioned rolled,
    2¼ cups
Paprika, ⅛ teaspoon
Pistachios, shelled, unsalted,
    2 tablespoons
Rosemary, dried, 2 teaspoons
Tomatoes crushed, no-salt-
    added, 1 (14.5 ounce) can
Vanilla extract, ½ teaspoon

MEATS AND SEAFOOD
Chicken breast, boneless,
    skinless, 2 (4-ounce)
Chicken breast tenders,
    1 pound
Pork tenderloin, 4 ounces
Trout, rainbow, 4 (4-ounce);
    use fillets if whole fish
    are unavailable

	BREAKFAST	SNACK	LUNCH	SNACK	PHYSICAL ACTIVITY	DINNER
SUNDAY	Black Bean Breakfast Bowl, page 51 (makes 2 servings)	1 serving fruit or vegetable (e.g., 1 apple or 1 cup baby carrots)	4 cups mixed salad greens with 4 ounces grilled fish, avocado slices	1 hardboiled egg with 1 cup baby carrots	Walk briskly for 30 minutes	Easy Herb-Baked Chicken Breasts, page 96 (makes 2 servings)
MONDAY	Leftover Black Bean Breakfast Bowl, page 51	1 serving fruit or vegetable (e.g., 1 apple or 1 cup baby carrots)	Leftover Easy Herb-Baked Chicken Breasts, page 96	1 cup low-fat Greek yogurt	Walk briskly for 30 minutes	Veggie Chili, page 85 (makes 4 servings; freeze 1 serving)
TUESDAY	1 slice whole-grain toast with 1 tablespoon nut butter, 6 ounces nonfat Greek yogurt, 1 banana	1 serving fruit or vegetable (e.g., 1 apple or 1 cup baby carrots)	Leftover Veggie Chili, page 85	1 ounce unsalted nuts with 1 medium piece of fruit	40 minutes of moderate-to-vigorous exercise	Shrimp Scampi with Spinach and Lemon, page 122 (makes 2 servings)
WEDNESDAY	Veggie Egg Mug, page 52 (makes 1 serving)	1 serving fruit or vegetable (e.g., 1 apple or 1 cup baby carrots)	Leftover Shrimp Scampi with Spinach and Lemon, page 122	½ cup low-fat cottage cheese with 1 medium piece of fruit	Walk briskly for 30 minutes	Southwestern Turkey-Quinoa Skillet, page 109 (makes 4 servings, freeze 1)
THURSDAY	Slow Cooker Grape, Walnut, and Banana Barley Breakfast Bowl, page 59 (makes 2 servings)	1 serving fruit or vegetable (e.g., 1 apple or 1 cup baby carrots)	Leftover Southwestern Turkey-Quinoa Skillet, page 109	1 cup low-fat plain Greek yogurt	Walk briskly for 30 minutes	4 ounces baked chicken breast, 1 cup steamed vegetables, ½ cup brown rice, green salad with olive oil
FRIDAY	1 cup oatmeal with 1 cup nonfat milk, 1 apple	1 serving fruit or vegetable (e.g., 1 apple or 1 cup baby carrots)	Leftover Veggie Chili, page 85	1 ounce unsalted nuts with 1 medium piece of fruit	Walk briskly for 30 minutes	Leftover Southwestern Turkey-Quinoa Skillet, page 109
SATURDAY	Leftover Slow Cooker Grape, Walnut, and Banana Barley Breakfast Bowl, page 59	1 serving fruit or vegetable (e.g., 1 apple or 1 cup baby carrots)	4 cups mixed salad greens with 4 ounces grilled chicken breast, avocado slices	1 low-fat string cheese with 1 medium piece of fruit	Walk briskly for 30 minutes	4 ounces grilled fish, 1 cup steamed vegetables, baked sweet potato, green salad with olive oil

Suggested Menu and Activity. Meals in blue are recipes from this book. Use the other meal suggestions as a guide, or swap them for recipes in this book. The physical activity can be done when it best suits your schedule, but aim to be active each day for at least 30 minutes.

Check your pantry and refrigerator for:

Almonds, raw, unsalted
Fresh fruit
Garlic
Milk, nonfat or low fat
Nonstick cooking spray
Oats, old-fashioned rolled

Olive oil
Onions
Peanut butter or other nut
   or seed butter, unsalted
Pepper
Salad greens, mixed

Salt
Sweetener of choice, such
   as stevia, pure maple
   syrup, honey
Vinegar of choice

Shop for:

FRESH PRODUCE: SNACKS
Fresh fruit and fresh vegetable: a combination of
   12 servings (you can also
   use canned fruit in light
   syrup or unsweetened dried
   fruit), including apples and
   baby carrots

FRESH PRODUCE: MEALS
Apple, 1
Avocados, 3
Bananas, 3
Basil or thyme, 1 small bunch
Carrots, baby, 1 cup
Garlic cloves, 6
Grapes, 1 bunch
Lemon, 1
Mushrooms, button, ½ cup
Onion, 1
Salad greens, mixed, 12 cups
   (about 30 ounces)
Shallots, 2
Spinach, baby, 5 cups
   (about 12 ounces)
Sweet potato, medium, 1
Tomatoes, cherry, 1 pint

FROZEN PRODUCE
Corn, 1 small (10-ounce)
   package
Mixed vegetables,
   1 (16-ounce) bag

GRAINS
Barley, hulled, ½ cup
Bread, whole-grain, 1 loaf
Pasta, angel hair,
   whole-wheat, 8 ounces
Quinoa, ½ cup
Rice, brown, ½ cup

DAIRY
Cottage cheese, low-fat
   1 small (8-ounce) container
Milk, nonfat, 1 cup
Parmesan cheese,
   grated, ¼ cup
String cheese, low-fat,
   1 string cheese
Yogurt, low-fat, Greek, 3 cups

EGGS
7 large

GROCERY ITEMS
Beans, black, 2 (15-ounce) cans
Beans, pinto, 2 (15-ounce) cans

Broth, vegetable,
   low-sodium, 1 cup
Chili powder, 2 tablespoons
Cinnamon, ground, 1 teaspoon
Corn, 1 (15-ounce) can
Cumin, ground, 2 teaspoons
Nut butter of choice, unsalted,
   1 tablespoon
Nut of choice, raw, unsalted,
   2 ounces
Oats, old-fashioned
   rolled, 1 cup
Red pepper flakes, ⅛ teaspoon
Tomatoes, chopped,
   fire-roasted, no-salt-added
   2 (14-ounce) cans
Walnuts, shelled,
   unsalted, ½ cup
Wine, white, dry,
   1 (750-mL) bottle

MEATS AND SEAFOOD
Chicken breast, boneless,
   skinless, 4 (4-ounce) pieces
Fish of choice,
   2 (4-ounce) fillets
Shrimp, large, peeled and
   deveined, 8 ounces
Turkey, 99% lean, ground,
   8 ounces

	BREAKFAST	SNACK	LUNCH	SNACK	PHYSICAL ACTIVITY	DINNER
SUNDAY	Baked Eggs in Avocado, page 53 (makes 2 servings)	1 serving fruit or vegetable (e.g., 1 apple or 1 cup baby carrots)	2 cups mixed salad greens, 4 ounces grilled fish, avocado slices	1 hardboiled egg with 1 cup baby carrots	Walk briskly for 30 minutes	Garlic-Ginger Chicken and Vegetable Stir-Fry, page 104 (makes 4 servings)
MONDAY	Leftover Baked Eggs in Avocado, page 53	1 serving fruit or vegetable (e.g., 1 apple or 1 cup baby carrots)	Leftover Garlic-Ginger Chicken and Vegetable Stir-Fry, page 104	1 cup low-fat Greek yogurt	Walk briskly for 30 minutes	Lentil and Spinach Stew, page 83 (makes 4 servings, freeze 1 serving)
TUESDAY	1 cup low-fat Greek yogurt, 1 banana, 2 tablespoons sliced almonds	1 serving fruit or vegetable (e.g., 1 apple or 1 cup baby carrots)	Leftover Garlic-Ginger Chicken and Vegetable Stir-Fry, page 104	1 ounce unsalted nuts with 1 medium piece of fruit	40 minutes of moderate-to-vigorous exercise	4 ounces grilled pork tenderloin, 1 cup steamed vegetables, ½ cup quinoa, mixed greens salad with olive oil and vinegar
WEDNESDAY	Steel-Cut Oats with Blueberries and Pecans, page 61 (makes 4 servings)	1 serving fruit or vegetable (e.g., 1 apple or 1 cup baby carrots)	Leftover Lentil and Spinach Stew, page 83	½ cup low-fat cottage cheese with 1 medium piece of fruit	Walk briskly for 30 minutes	Leftover Garlic-Ginger Chicken and Vegetable Stir-Fry, page 104
THURSDAY	Leftover Steel-Cut Oats with Blueberries and Pecans, page 61	1 serving fruit or vegetable (e.g., 1 apple or 1 cup baby carrots)	2 cups mixed salad greens, 4 ounces grilled chicken breast, avocado slices	1 cup low-fat Greek yogurt	Walk briskly for 30 minutes	Slow Cooker Turkey and Chickpea Chili, page 105 (makes 6 servings, freeze 3 servings)
FRIDAY	Leftover Steel-Cut Oats with Blueberries and Pecans, page 61	1 serving fruit or vegetable (e.g., 1 apple or 1 cup baby carrots)	Leftover Lentil and Spinach Stew, page 83	1 ounce unsalted nuts with 1 medium piece of fruit	Walk briskly for 30 minutes	Leftover Slow Cooker Turkey and Chickpea Chili, page 105
SATURDAY	Leftover Steel-Cut Oats with Blueberries and Pecans, page 61	1 serving fruit or vegetable (e.g., 1 apple or 1 cup baby carrots)	Leftover Slow Cooker Turkey and Chickpea Chili, page 105	1 low-fat string cheese with 1 medium piece of fruit	40 minutes of moderate-to-vigorous exercise	4 ounces grilled fish, 1 cup steamed vegetables, baked sweet potato, green salad, avocado slices

Suggested Menu and Activity. Meals in blue are recipes from this book. Use the other meal suggestions as a guide, or swap them for recipes in this book. The physical activity can be done when it suits your schedule the best, but aim to be active each day for at least 30 minutes.

Check your pantry and refrigerator for:

Almonds, raw, unsalted
Fresh fruit
Garlic
Milk, nonfat or low fat
Nonstick cooking spray
Oats, old-fashioned rolled

Olive oil
Onions
Peanut butter or other nut
    or seed butter, unsalted
Pepper
Salad greens, mixed

Salt
Sweetener of choice,
    such as stevia, pure
    maple syrup, honey
Vinegar of choice

Shop for:

FRESH PRODUCE: SNACKS
Fresh fruit and fresh vege-
    tables: a combination of
    12 servings (you can also
    use canned fruit in light
    syrup or unsweetened dried
    fruit), including apples and
    baby carrots

FRESH PRODUCE: MEALS
Avocados, 3 large
Banana, 1
Blueberries, 1 pint
Cilantro, 1 small bunch
Garlic cloves, 13
Ginger, 1 (2-inch) piece
Mushrooms, portobello,
    3 medium
Salad greens, mixed, 8 cups
    (about 20 ounces)
Sweet potato, 1 medium

FROZEN PRODUCE
Mixed vegetables,
    1 (16-ounce) package
Spinach, 2 (10-ounce)
    packages

Stir-fry vegetables,
    1 (16-ounce) package

GRAINS
Quinoa, ½ cup

DAIRY
Cottage cheese, low-fat
    1 small (8-ounce) container
Milk, nonfat or low-fat, 2 cups
String cheese, low-fat,
    1 string cheese
Yogurt, low-fat Greek, 3 cups

EGGS
3 large

GROCERY ITEMS
Almonds, unsalted, sliced,
    2 tablespoons
Broth, chicken,
    low-sodium, 2 cups
Brown sugar, 2 tablespoons
Chickpeas, 1 (15-ounce) can
Chili powder, 1 tablespoon
Cumin, ground, 1 teaspoon

Green chilies, diced
    1 (6-ounce) can
Lentils, green, 1 cup
Nut of choice, raw, unsalted,
    2 ounces
Oats, steel-cut, 1 cup
Oil, sesame, 1 tablespoon
Pecans, raw, shelled,
    unsalted, ¼ cup
Soy sauce, low-sodium,
    2 tablespoons
Sweet potato, 1 medium
Tomatoes, diced, no-salt-
    added, 2 (14-ounce) cans
Tomato paste, no-salt-added,
    1 (6-ounce) can

MEATS AND SEAFOOD
Chicken breast, boneless,
    skinless, 1 (4-ounce) piece
    plus 1 pound boneless,
    skinless breasts or tenders
Fish of choice,
    2 (4-ounce) fillets
Pork tenderloin, 4 ounces
Turkey breast, boneless,
    skinless, 1½ pounds

	BREAKFAST	SNACK	LUNCH	SNACK	PHYSICAL ACTIVITY	DINNER
SUNDAY	Sweet Potato Toast with Avocado-Chickpea Spread, page 50 (makes 2 servings)	1 serving fruit or vegetable (e.g., 1 apple or 1 cup baby carrots)	4 ounces grilled chicken breast, 1 cup steamed vegetables, ½ cup brown rice	1 hardboiled egg with 1 cup baby carrots	Walk briskly for 30 minutes	Yogurt-Marinated Grilled Salmon, page 116 (makes 4 servings)
MONDAY	Leftover Sweet Potato Toast with Avocado-Chickpea Spread, page 50	1 serving fruit or vegetable (e.g., 1 apple or 1 cup baby carrots)	Leftover Yogurt-Marinated Grilled Salmon, page 116 over 2 cups mixed salad greens	1 cup low-fat plain Greek yogurt	40 minutes of moderate-to-vigorous exercise	Garlicky Black Bean Soup, page 84 (makes 4 servings, freeze 1)
TUESDAY	Banana-Oat Pancakes, page 56 (makes 2 servings)	1 serving fruit or vegetable (e.g., 1 apple or 1 cup baby carrots)	Leftover Garlicky Black Bean Soup, page 84	1 ounce unsalted nuts with 1 medium piece of fruit	Walk briskly for 30 minutes	Chicken and Zucchini Burgers, page 97 (makes 4 servings, freeze 2)
WEDNESDAY	Bowl of oat cereal with low-fat milk, 6 ounces Greek yogurt, fresh berries	1 serving fruit or vegetable (e.g., 1 apple or 1 cup baby carrots)	Leftover Garlicky Black Bean Soup, page 84	½ cup low-fat cottage cheese with 1 medium piece of fruit	40 minutes of moderate-to-vigorous exercise	Leftover Yogurt-Marinated Grilled Salmon, page 116 with Easy Roasted Asparagus, page 156
THURSDAY	Leftover Banana-Oat Pancakes, page 56	1 serving fruit or vegetable (e.g., 1 apple or 1 cup baby carrots)	Leftover Chicken and Zucchini Burgers, page 97	1 cup low-fat plain Greek yogurt	Walk briskly for 30 minutes	4 ounces grilled beef tenderloin, 1 cup mixed vegetables, ½ cup barley
FRIDAY	1 cup oatmeal with 1 cup nonfat milk, 1 apple	1 serving fruit or vegetable (e.g., 1 apple or 1 cup baby carrots)	Leftover Garlicky Black Bean Soup, page 84	1 ounce unsalted nuts with 1 medium piece of fruit	Walk briskly for 30 minutes	Leftover Yogurt-Marinated Grilled Salmon, page 116 with Parsnip Fries, page 161
SATURDAY	Whole-grain toast with 1 tablespoon nut butter, 6 ounces low-fat Greek yogurt, 1 piece fruit	1 serving fruit or vegetable (e.g., 1 apple or 1 cup baby carrots)	Leftover Chicken and Zucchini Burgers, page 97	1 low-fat string cheese with 1 medium piece of fruit	40 minutes of moderate-to-vigorous exercise	4 ounces grilled pork tenderloin, 1 cup steamed vegetables, baked sweet potato, mixed greens salad with olive oil and vinegar, avocado slices

Suggested Menu and Activity. Meals in blue are recipes from this book. Use the other meal suggestions as a guide, or swap them for recipes in this book. The physical activity can be done when it suits your schedule the best, but aim to be active each day for at least 30 minutes.

Check your pantry and refrigerator for:

Almonds, raw, unsalted
Fresh fruit
Garlic
Milk, nonfat or low fat
Nonstick cooking spray
Oats, old-fashioned rolled

Olive oil
Onions
Peanut butter or other nut
    or seed butter, unsalted
Pepper
Salad greens, mixed

Salt
Sweetener of choice, such
    as stevia, pure maple
    syrup, honey
Vinegar of choice

Shop for:

FRESH PRODUCE: SNACKS
Fresh fruit and fresh vege-
    tables: a combination of
    12 servings (you can also
    use canned fruit in light
    syrup or unsweetened dried
    fruit), including apples and
    baby carrots

FRESH PRODUCE: MEALS
Apple, 1
Asparagus, 2 pounds
Avocados, 2
Baby carrots, 1 cup
Bananas, 2 medium
Berries, fresh, any type, 1 pint
Cilantro, 1 bunch
Garlic cloves, 6
Lemons, 2
Onion, 1 small
Parsnips, 2 pounds
Rosemary, 1 bunch
Salad greens, mixed, 2 cups
    (about 5 ounces)
Scallions, 2
Sweet potatoes, 3 medium
Tomato, 1 medium
Zucchini, 1 medium

FROZEN PRODUCE:
Mixed vegetables,
    2 (16-ounce) packages

GRAINS:
Barley, hulled, ½ cup
Bread, whole-grain, 1 loaf
Rice, brown, ½ cup

DAIRY:
Cottage cheese, low-fat,
    1 small (8-ounce) container
Milk, nonfat or low-fat, 2 cups
String cheese, low-fat,
    1 string cheese
Yogurt, low-fat Greek,
    4½ cups

EGGS:
4 large

GROCERY ITEMS:
Baking powder, ½ teaspoon
Beans, black,
    2 (15-ounce) cans
Bread crumbs, panko,
    whole-wheat, ½ cup

Cereal, oat, 1 box
Chickpeas, 1 (15-ounce) can
Cumin, ground, 1 teaspoon
Lemon juice, 1 bottle
Maple syrup or honey, for
    serving with pancakes
Nut butter of choice, unsalted,
    1 tablespoon
Nut of choice, raw, unsalted,
    2 ounces
Oats, old-fashioned rolled,
    1½ cups
Sriracha, 1 tablespoon
Tomatoes, diced, fire-roasted,
    no-salt-added,
    1 (14-ounce) can

MEATS AND SEAFOOD:
Beef tenderloin, 4 ounces
Chicken breast, boneless,
    skinless 4 ounces
Chicken, lean, white meat,
    ground, 1 pound
Pork tenderloin, 4 ounces
Salmon fillets, boneless,
    skinless, 4 (4-ounce)

PART TWO

....

LOW-CHOLESTEROL RECIPES

All recipes in this book yield from one to four servings, and use readily available ingredients that are both nutritious and economical. Recipes are high in soluble and insoluble fiber, vitamins, and minerals, antioxidants, and low in saturated fat, trans fats, sodium, and added sugars. The recipe ingredients have been selected for their cholesterol-lowering properties, including sources of pectin and soluble fiber; phytonutrients from garlic, onions, and shallots; and heart-healthy fats and fiber from avocado and nuts, among numerous other nutritious foods.

Recipe labels will help you quickly learn more about each recipe's attributes. Labels include:

5 MAIN INGREDIENTS	The recipe is made using 5 main ingredients not including salt, pepper, or oils.
30 MINUTES OR FEWER	The recipes can be prepared in 30 minutes or fewer.
BUDGET SAVER	A budget saver recipe costs $5 to $10 to make, and allows for the use of frozen, canned, and dried ingredients.
DAIRY FREE	The recipe does not contain any milk products, but may include eggs.
LOW SODIUM	The recipe has less than 500 mg of sodium per serving.
NUT FREE	The recipe does not contain any nuts.
ONE POT	The recipes require only one pot or one sheet pan to cook.

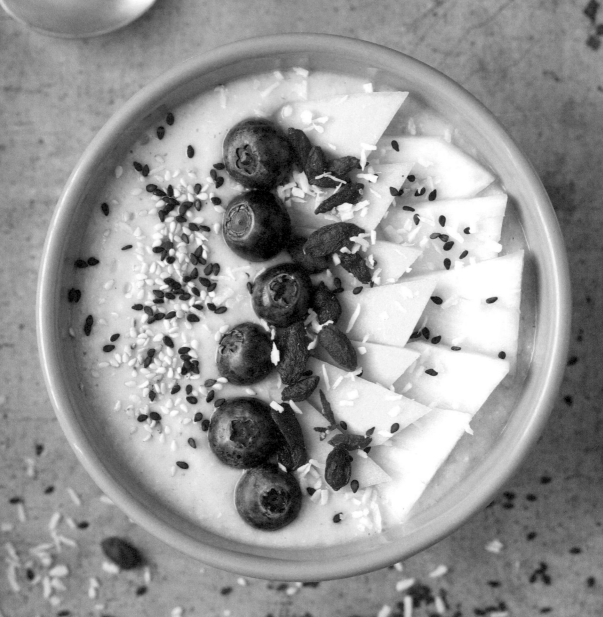

CHAPTER 4

Breakfasts and Smoothies

Blueberry, Oat, and Almond Smoothie

Serves 2 | Prep time: 5 minutes

➤ **PER SERVING** CALORIES: 347; TOTAL FAT: 10G; SATURATED FAT: 0G; TRANS FAT: 0G; CHOLESTEROL: 5MG; SODIUM: 91MG; TOTAL CARBOHYDRATE: 54G; FIBER: 8G; SUGAR: 29G; PROTEIN: 16G

A low-cholesterol diet should be full of colorful and nutrient-dense foods that lower LDL cholesterol while satisfying your cravings and tasting delicious. Smoothies are a quick and convenient way to enjoy a nutritious breakfast with little prep. Creamy and sweet, this recipe is high in soluble fiber from oats, antioxidants from blueberries, and healthy unsaturated fats from almonds. Almond butter is used here for its cholesterol-lowering qualities, but feel free to substitute another nut butter if you like.

1 cup nonfat vanilla Greek yogurt

1 cup frozen blueberries

2 tablespoons almond butter

1 frozen banana, sliced

½ cup old-fashioned rolled oats

¾ water

1 cup ice

1 In a high-speed blender, combine the yogurt, blueberries, almond butter, banana, and oats. Process until smooth.

2 Add the water and ice, a little bit at a time, and blend until you achieve your desired consistency. Serve immediately.

Did you know? Frozen bananas are a "secret ingredient" for making smoothies that are both thick and creamy. For an added bonus, bananas are rich in soluble fiber, the type of fiber that removes cholesterol from your bloodstream. Keep a bag of sliced bananas in your freezer so you have them on hand.

5 MAIN INGREDIENTS	30 MINUTES OR FEWER	BUDGET SAVER	LOW SODIUM	ONE POT	

Strawberry-Raspberry Yogurt Smoothie

Serves 2 | Prep time: 5 minutes

> ➤ PER SERVING   CALORIES: 217; TOTAL FAT: 3G; SATURATED FAT: 0G; TRANS FAT: 0G; CHOLESTEROL: 5MG; SODIUM: 37MG; TOTAL CARBOHYDRATE: 39G; FIBER: 9G; SUGAR: 24G; PROTEIN: 11G

Berries have great benefits for heart health, and strawberries, in particular, are high in antioxidants and contain a unique protein that works to lower both triglycerides and LDL cholesterol. With added fiber from raspberries and probiotic-rich yogurt, this cholesterol-busting smoothie is also sweet and delicious.

1 cup frozen strawberries

1 cup frozen raspberries

1 cup nonfat vanilla Greek yogurt, or traditional-style yogurt

2 tablespoons ground flaxseed

½ frozen banana, sliced

¾ cup water

1 cup ice

1 In a high-speed blender, combine the strawberries, raspberries, yogurt, flaxseed, and banana. Process until smooth.

2 Add the water and ice, a little bit at a time, and blend until you achieve your desired consistency. Serve immediately.

Substitution tip To make this dairy-free, substitute an equal amount of silken tofu for the yogurt. Consuming 25 grams of soy protein a day (10 ounces of tofu or 2½ cups soy milk) can lower LDL cholesterol by 5 to 6 percent.

	5 MAIN INGREDIENTS	30 MINUTES OR FEWER	BUDGET SAVER	LOW SODIUM	NUT FREE	ONE POT	

Avocado-Apple Green Smoothie

Serves 2 | Prep time: 5 minutes

➤ **PER SERVING** CALORIES: 319; TOTAL FAT: 16G; SATURATED FAT: 2G; TRANS FAT: 0G; CHOLESTEROL: 0MG; SODIUM: 128MG; TOTAL CARBOHYDRATE: 43G; FIBER: 11G; SUGAR: 25G; PROTEIN: 9G

This dairy-free, creamy green smoothie is packed with cholesterol-lowering ingredients and protein to keep you feeling full. Apple, avocado, and orange all contain significant amounts of dietary fiber, which may reduce LDL cholesterol and boost heart health. Soy milk adds protein and beneficial plant antioxidants to make this a balanced, nutrient-rich, super speedy breakfast.

2 cups plain low-fat soy milk

2 cups fresh baby spinach (optional)

1 large Granny Smith apple, chilled, cored, and sliced

1 navel orange, peeled and frozen (see tip)

1 ripe avocado, peeled, pitted, and cubed

½ frozen ripe banana, sliced

1 cup ice, or as needed

1 In a high-speed blender, combine the soy milk, spinach (if using), apple, orange, avocado, and banana. Process until smooth.

2 Add the ice, a little bit at a time, and blend until you achieve your desired consistency. Serve immediately.

Ingredient tip Freezing the orange before blending gives the smoothie a thicker texture. Using it fresh gives it a stronger citrus flavor.

5 MAIN INGREDIENTS	30 MINUTES OR FEWER	BUDGET SAVER	DAIRY FREE	LOW SODIUM	NUT FREE	ONE POT

Tropical Smoothie Bowl

Serves 2 | Prep time: 10 minutes

➤ PER SERVING   CALORIES: 252; TOTAL FAT: 6G; SATURATED FAT: 4G; TRANS FAT: 0G; CHOLESTEROL: 9MG; SODIUM: 62MG; TOTAL CARBOHYDRATE: 49G; FIBER: 6G; SUGAR: 33G; PROTEIN: 7G

This tropical-inspired smoothie bowl is a cool, creamy, and creative way to change up the traditional smoothie. A perfect way to get more fruit and plant-based foods into your diet, smoothie bowls are meant to be thicker so you can eat them out of a bowl with a spoon. The toppings let you add even more flavors and textures to create a filling breakfast that will transport you to the island . . . at least in your dreams.

FOR THE SMOOTHIE BOWLS

1 cup unsweetened coconut milk

½ cup plain low-fat Greek yogurt

1 frozen banana, cut into chunks

1 cup frozen mango

FOR THE TOPPINGS

½ cup fresh blueberries

½ cup fresh pineapple wedges

½ cup fresh mango wedges

2 teaspoons unsweetened
   shredded coconut

2 tablespoons goji berries, hemp seeds,
   or sesame seeds (optional)

TO MAKE THE SMOOTHIE BOWLS

1 In a high-speed blender, combine the coconut milk, yogurt, banana, and mango. Blend to your desired consistency.

2 Divide between two serving bowls and top each with ¼ cup of blueberries, ¼ cup of pineapple, ¼ cup of mango, and 1 teaspoon of coconut. Add optional toppings as desired. Enjoy.

	30 MINUTES OR FEWER	BUDGET SAVER	LOW SODIUM	ONE POT	

Sweet Potato Toast with Avocado-Chickpea Spread

Serves 2 | **Prep time: 5 minutes** | **Cook time: 10 minutes**

➤ **PER SERVING** CALORIES: 348; TOTAL FAT: 9G; SATURATED FAT: 1G; TRANS FAT: 0G; CHOLESTEROL: 0MG; SODIUM: 30MG; TOTAL CARBOHYDRATE: 60G; FIBER: 13G; SUGAR: 9G; PROTEIN: 10G

Sweet potatoes are one of the best soluble fiber–rich foods you can include in your cholesterol-lowering diet. An excellent source of vitamin A in the form of beta-carotene, the sweet potato is also a good source of vitamin C and heart-healthy potassium and B vitamins. This healthy, crunchy recipe uses sweet potato slices for bread, topped with a delicious avocado-chickpea spread to create a power-packed breakfast loaded with nutrients.

2 medium sweet potatoes, washed, peel on, cut lengthwise into ¼-inch-thick slices

1 cup canned chickpeas, drained and rinsed

½ ripe avocado, mashed

1 teaspoon freshly squeezed lemon juice

Freshly ground black pepper

1 medium tomato, sliced

Pinch salt (optional)

1 Place the sweet potato slices in a microwave-safe dish and microwave on high power for 30 seconds.

2 Turn your toaster to high and toast each sweet potato slice two to three times until browned and crispy, similar to toasted bread, about 8 minutes.

3 In a small bowl, mash the chickpeas with a fork. Add the mashed avocado and stir to combine.

4 Stir in the lemon juice and season with pepper. Divide the mash among the toasted sweet potato slices.

5 Top with tomato slices, season with salt (if using), and serve.

Ingredient tip Choose large round sweet potatoes, as you can get the best slices from them. You don't have to peel the sweet potatoes (the peel is rich in fiber and antioxidants), but you can if you prefer.

5 MAIN INGREDIENTS	30 MINUTES OR FEWER	BUDGET SAVER	DAIRY FREE	LOW SODIUM	NUT FREE

Black Bean Breakfast Bowl

Serves 2 | Prep time: 10 minutes | Cook time: 6 minutes

➤ **PER SERVING** CALORIES: 459; TOTAL FAT: 25G; SATURATED FAT: 4G; TRANS FAT: 0G; CHOLESTEROL: 186MG; SODIUM: 85MG; TOTAL CARBOHYDRATE: 42G; FIBER: 15G; SUGAR: 2G; PROTEIN: 19G

The concept of "bowl" recipes is to combine a high-fiber carbohydrate, plus a protein, plus veggies to create a healthy dish served in one bowl. This recipe features protein- and fiber-rich black beans for slow-burning carbs, eggs for vitamin D and protein, avocado for healthy fats and more cholesterol-lowering fiber, and tomatoes for antioxidants. Versatile and quick to prepare, this recipe can be customized with your favorites.

1 tablespoon olive oil

2 large eggs, beaten

1 (15-ounce) can black beans, drained and rinsed

1 teaspoon ground cumin

1 avocado, peeled, pitted, and diced

10 cherry tomatoes, halved

Freshly ground black pepper

1 In a small pan over medium heat, heat the olive oil.

2 Add the eggs, and cook for 3 to 5 minutes, stirring, until set.

3 Place the black beans in a microwave-safe bowl and season with the cumin. Heat on high power for about 1 minute until warm. Divide the warmed beans between two bowls.

4 Top each bowl with half each of the scrambled eggs, avocado, and cherry tomatoes. Season with pepper and serve.

Substitution tip If you want a vegan breakfast bowl, swap the eggs for tofu to create a quick tofu and black bean bowl. You can also add more veggies, such as spinach and mushrooms, mix up the spices in the black beans, or swap black beans for chickpeas.

	5 MAIN INGREDIENTS	30 MINUTES OR FEWER	BUDGET SAVER	DAIRY FREE	LOW SODIUM	NUT FREE	

Veggie Egg Mug

Serves 1 | Prep time: 5 minutes | Cook time: 4 minutes

➤ **PER SERVING** CALORIES: 141; TOTAL FAT: 5G; SATURATED FAT: 1G; TRANS FAT: 0G; CHOLESTEROL: 0MG; SODIUM: 237MG; TOTAL CARBOHYDRATE: 9G; FIBER: 3G; SUGAR: 4G; PROTEIN: 17G

Microwave egg mugs are a quick and easy way to power up for a busy day. Fresh baby spinach, mushrooms, onions, and avocado add vitamins, minerals, fiber, and healthy fats to this protein-packed breakfast. You can try your favorite veggies, herbs, and seasonings to create other healthy combinations.

Olive oil mister, or nonstick
   cooking spray
½ cup chopped fresh baby spinach
½ cup sliced button mushrooms
¼ cup thinly sliced onion
4 large egg whites
2 tablespoons diced avocado
Freshly ground black pepper

1 Spray a large microwave-safe mug (at least 16 ounces, or use a 2-cup glass measuring cup) with your olive oil mister or cooking spray. Add the spinach, mushrooms, and onion. Cook on high power for 2 minutes, or until softened.

2 Add the egg whites, stir, and microwave for 1 minute. Stir, microwave for about 30 seconds longer, or until the egg whites are set.

3 Top with avocado, season with pepper, and enjoy!

Ingredient tip Depending on the mug used, the eggs may rise up over the top, but won't overflow. They deflate quickly once the mug is removed from the microwave.

5 MAIN INGREDIENTS	30 MINUTES OR FEWER	BUDGET SAVER	DAIRY FREE	LOW SODIUM	NUT FREE	ONE POT

Baked Eggs in Avocado

Serves 2 | Prep time: 5 minutes | Cook time: 22 minutes

➤ **PER SERVING** CALORIES: 239; TOTAL FAT: 18G; SATURATED FAT: 4G; TRANS FAT: 0G; CHOLESTEROL: 186MG; SODIUM: 83MG; TOTAL CARBOHYDRATE: 13G; FIBER: 7G; SUGAR: 1G; PROTEIN: 9G

Avocados are full of healthy monounsaturated fats and potassium, and may help lower cholesterol and triglyceride levels due to their large amount of dietary fiber. Used in this quick and easy recipe, hollowed-out avocados are baked with eggs, garlic, and tomato. Consuming garlic on a daily basis may help lower cholesterol levels due to the antioxidant properties of allicin—if you're a garlic lover, add it to recipes whenever you can.

1 large avocado, halved and pitted

2 large eggs

4 garlic cloves, sliced

6 cherry tomatoes, sliced

6 fresh cilantro leaves for serving

Salt

Freshly ground black pepper

1 Preheat the oven or toaster oven to 450°F.

2 Scoop out 2 tablespoons of avocado flesh from the center of each avocado half to make room for the eggs.

3 Place the avocado halves in a tight-fitting ovenproof bowl. Crack one egg into each avocado half.

4 Top each with garlic and tomatoes. Bake for 20 to 22 minutes, until the eggs are set. Serve garnished with cilantro and seasoned with salt and pepper.

Ingredient tip Store avocados at room temperature until they are fully ripe. You can speed up their ripening by placing them in a brown paper bag. If the avocado yields to light pressure, it's ready to use. After they are cut, sprinkle a small amount of lemon or lime juice on the exposed flesh to help cut down on discoloration, wrap tightly in plastic wrap, and refrigerate.

If you have trouble finding the perfect avocado, there are a couple of tricks you can use: First look at the color: a deeper green usually means a riper avocado. Second, feel the firmness and try to find one that is soft to the touch but not mushy. Last, pop off the brown stem and check the color: If you see a nice shade of green, the avocado is ripe.

5 MAIN INGREDIENTS	30 MINUTES OR FEWER	BUDGET SAVER	DAIRY FREE	LOW SODIUM	NUT FREE	ONE POT

Kale and Sweet Potato Hash

Serves 4 | Prep time: 10 minutes | Cook time: 10 minutes

➤ **PER SERVING** CALORIES: 228; TOTAL FAT: 13G; SATURATED FAT: 3G; TRANS FAT: 0G; CHOLESTEROL: 186MG; SODIUM: 129MG; TOTAL CARBOHYDRATE: 19G; FIBER: 4G; SUGAR: 3G; PROTEIN: 10G

This one-pot breakfast hash features a number of colorful and delicious foods with cholesterol-lowering abilities. Allicin from garlic, phytosterols from pumpkin seeds, and fiber and antioxidants from kale and sweet potatoes combine to give this dish extraordinary nutrition to boost your heart health, while providing long-lasting energy. Feel free to swap out the kale for your favorite green, such as fresh baby spinach, collards, or Swiss chard. All greens are nutrient dense with valuable amounts of soluble fiber, vitamins, and minerals. This recipe also makes a perfect lunch or dinner.

2 tablespoons olive oil

6 garlic cloves, chopped

1 cup diced sweet potato
 (about 1 medium)

4 cups coarsely chopped kale
 (see tip)

¼ cup water

4 large eggs, whisked

¼ teaspoon freshly ground
 black pepper

¼ cup shelled pumpkin seeds

1 In a medium nonstick pan over medium heat, heat the olive oil.

2 Add the garlic, sweet potatoes, and kale. Sauté for 2 minutes, until the garlic becomes fragrant.

3 Add the water and loosely cover the pan. Reduce the heat to medium-low and simmer for 5 minutes, until the potatoes soften and the kale is tender.

4 Remove the lid and add the eggs. Cook for about 3 minutes, stirring gently, until the eggs are cooked through. Serve seasoned with pepper and sprinkled with pumpkin seeds.

Ingredient tip When cooking kale, it's best to use a skillet with high sides (a wok works well, too) as the volume may be overwhelming at first, but the high sides help keep things contained. The kale quickly wilts and becomes manageable, and it is possible to continue to feed the pan with handfuls of fresh kale as it wilts and more room is created.

5 MAIN INGREDIENTS	30 MINUTES OR FEWER	DAIRY FREE	LOW SODIUM	NUT FREE	ONE POT

Cranberry-Orange Muffin in a Mug

Serves 1 | Prep time: 3 minutes | Cook time: 1 minute

➤ **PER SERVING**   CALORIES: 335; TOTAL FAT: 15G; SATURATED FAT: 3G; TRANS FAT: 0G; CHOLESTEROL: 187MG; SODIUM: 324MG; TOTAL CARBOHYDRATE: 37G; FIBER: 7G; SUGAR: 6G; PROTEIN: 17G

If you are trying to lower your cholesterol, you probably know that the muffins you buy at coffee shops or bakeries are high in calories, sugar, salt, and often unhealthy fats. Skip the trip and make your own much healthier muffin in less time than it takes to park your car at a coffee shop. This single-serve muffin is high in fiber, antioxidants, and protein; offers instant portion control; and tastes delicious!

1 large egg

2 tablespoons nonfat vanilla Greek yogurt

1 tablespoon nut butter of choice (cashew butter or peanut butter both work great)

1 tablespoon oat flour, or whole-wheat pastry flour

¼ cup old-fashioned rolled oats

½ teaspoon baking powder

Pinch salt

¼ cup fresh cranberries

½ navel orange, peeled and chopped

Nonstick cooking spray

1 In a medium bowl, beat the egg.

2 Stir in the yogurt and nut butter and mix well.

3 Add the flour, oats, baking powder, and salt. Stir until thoroughly mixed.

4 Gently stir in the cranberries and orange.

5 Spray a 16-ounce mug with the cooking spray. Spoon the batter into the mug. Microwave for 45 to 55 seconds on high power, or until set. Enjoy immediately.

Substitution tip Instead of cranberry and orange, try blueberry and banana, or create your own fruit combinations based on your favorites.

30 MINUTES OR FEWER	BUDGET SAVER	LOW SODIUM	ONE POT

Banana-Oat Pancakes

Serves 2 | Prep time: 5 minutes | Cook time: 15 minutes

➤ **PER SERVING** CALORIES: 253; TOTAL FAT: 7G; SATURATED FAT: 2G; TRANS FAT: 0G; CHOLESTEROL: 186MG; SODIUM: 194MG; TOTAL CARBOHYDRATE: 41G; FIBER: 5G; SUGAR: 15G; PROTEIN: 10G

These easy flourless pancakes are made with old-fashioned rolled oats and bananas, two foods rich in cholesterol-lowering fiber. With no added chemicals or fillers, this nutritious recipe makes a filling and healthy breakfast.

2 medium bananas

2 large eggs

½ cup old-fashioned rolled oats

½ teaspoon baking powder

Pinch salt

Nonstick cooking spray

Fresh fruit of choice, for serving

Pure maple syrup or honey, for serving
(optional)

1 In a blender or food processor, combine the bananas, eggs, oats, baking powder, and salt. Blend until the mixture is smooth and blended well, 1 to 2 minutes depending on your blender's power. Let the batter stand for 10 minutes until thickened slightly.

2 Heat a nonstick skillet over medium heat. Lightly spray it with cooking spray.

3 Drop 2-tablespoonful portions of batter into the skillet and fry until golden brown on both sides, about 4 minutes per side.

4 Serve with fresh fruit and a drizzle of maple syrup or honey (if using).

	5 MAIN INGREDIENTS	30 MINUTES OR FEWER	BUDGET SAVER	DAIRY FREE	LOW SODIUM	NUT FREE	

No-Bake Almond Butter and Oatmeal Breakfast Bars

Makes 20 bars | Prep time: 5 minutes | Cook time: 1 minute, plus 4 hours chilling

➤ **PER SERVING (1 BAR)** CALORIES: 128; TOTAL FAT: 7G; SATURATED FAT: 1G; TRANS FAT: 0G; CHOLESTEROL: 0MG; SODIUM: 4MG; TOTAL CARBOHYDRATE: 14G; FIBER: 3G; SUGAR: 4G; PROTEIN: 4G

These soft, chewy bars are easy to make for a naturally sweet and healthy breakfast. Packed with soluble fiber, protein, and healthy fats, making your own bars from scratch rather than buying processed foods ensures you don't get unwanted sodium, chemicals, and unhealthy fats. A great batch recipe, pair these bars with a piece of fruit and some yogurt or a glass of milk for a quick grab-and-go breakfast.

Nonstick cooking spray

1 cup almond butter, or other
   nut butter of choice

¼ cup pure maple syrup

3 cups old-fashioned rolled oats

¼ cup unsweetened vanilla almond
   milk, or nonfat milk

1 Line a 9-by-9-inch pan with aluminum foil and lightly spray it with cooking spray.

2 In a medium microwave-safe dish, stir together the almond butter and maple syrup. Cook for 30 seconds on high power, stir, and cook for 30 seconds more.

3 Add the oats and almond milk. Stir until combined. Press the oat mixture into the prepared pan. Refrigerate or freeze for about 4 hours, until the bars are set and somewhat hard to the touch.

4 Lift the foil to remove the bars from the pan and cut into 20 bars. Refrigerate in an airtight container until ready to serve.

5 MAIN INGREDIENTS	DAIRY FREE	LOW SODIUM

Homemade Granola

Serves 6 | Prep time: 10 minutes | Cook time: 10 minutes

➤ **PER SERVING (½ CUP)** CALORIES: 261; TOTAL FAT: 12G; SATURATED FAT: 1G; TRANS FAT: 0G; CHOLESTEROL: 0MG; SODIUM: 16MG; TOTAL CARBOHYDRATE: 34G; FIBER: 5G; SUGAR: 10G; PROTEIN: 7G

Who doesn't love granola? It makes a great breakfast, a tasty snack, and a perfect topping for parfaits and smoothie bowls. But store-bought granolas are typically very high in unhealthy fats, sugar, and salt—and loaded with calories. The good news is, it is easy to make your own granola, and this recipe was created to be especially rich in foods with cholesterol-lowering properties. This recipe uses oat bran, which is the outer husk of the oat grain that contains the bulk of its dietary fiber. You can find oat bran with the other hot cereals at your local grocery, or in the bulk aisle. Add it to smoothies, cookies, muffins, and breads. Oat bran and wheat bran are not the same thing, so be sure to clarify when buying at your local grocery store.

2 cups old-fashioned rolled oats

1 cup unsweetened dried apple

⅓ cup oat bran (see headnote)

½ cup chopped raw, unsalted almonds

¼ cup raw, shelled pumpkin seeds

2 to 3 tablespoons pure maple syrup, or honey

1 tablespoon plus 1 teaspoon avocado oil, or canola oil

½ teaspoon vanilla extract, or almond extract

Pinch salt

1 Preheat the oven to 300°F.

2 In a large bowl, combine the oats, dried apple, oat bran, almonds, pumpkin seeds, maple syrup, avocado oil, vanilla, and salt. Using your clean hands, mix everything well and toss to coat—it will be sticky and messy. Spread the mixture into a thin layer on a baking sheet and bake for 10 minutes until very lightly toasted. (It may help to use wax paper to thinly spread the mixture.)

3 Cool completely before serving or storing in an airtight container in a cool, dry place for up to 2 weeks.

Ingredient tip This recipe uses avocado oil in place of olive oil, because olive oil tends to have a strong flavor. While avocado oil is not as well known as olive oil, it's just as delicious, versatile, and easy to incorporate into your diet. Super easy to find and priced comparably to olive oil, your local Walmart stocks it with the other cooking oils. If you can't find avocado oil, you can use canola oil instead.

	30 MINUTES OR FEWER	DAIRY FREE	LOW SODIUM	

Slow Cooker Grape, Walnut, and Banana Barley Breakfast Bowl

Serves 2 | Prep time: 5 minutes | Cook time: 8 hours or overnight

➤ **PER SERVING**   CALORIES: 392; TOTAL FAT: 11G; SATURATED FAT: 1G; TRANS FAT: 0G; CHOLESTEROL: 0MG; SODIUM: 3MG; TOTAL CARBOHYDRATE: 71G; FIBER: 11G; SUGAR: 21G; PROTEIN: 9G

When it comes to cholesterol-lowering grains, oats are always in the spotlight. However, hulled barley deserves a place on your plate, too, as unrefined barley is the single best food source of beta glucan, the same soluble fiber found in oats that can lower cholesterol. Rich in pectin, another soluble fiber, hulled barley takes longer to cook than refined pearl barley, so this recipe uses a slow cooker. With added cholesterol-lowering nutrients from grapes, bananas, and walnuts, prep this at night and wake up to a hot, heart-healthy breakfast.

3 cups water

½ cup hulled barley (not pearl or quick-cooking pearl)

2 bananas, sliced

1 teaspoon ground cinnamon

½ cup grapes, sliced, for topping

¼ cup chopped walnuts, for topping

1 In a 2-quart slow cooker, combine the water, barley, bananas, and cinnamon. Cover and cook for about 8 hours on low heat.

2 Serve topped with grapes and walnuts.

Ingredient tip You can also make this on the stove top using a 1:3 ratio of barley to water. Bring the water to a boil. Add the barley, reduce the heat to low, cover, and cook for 45 to 50 minutes. The barley is done when it has tripled in volume and is soft yet chewy. Fluff with a fork and serve.

5 MAIN INGREDIENTS	BUDGET SAVER	DAIRY FREE	LOW SODIUM	ONE POT

Pear-Pistachio Overnight Oats

Serves 2 | Prep time: 5 minutes | Chill time: overnight

➤ **PER SERVING**   CALORIES: 271; TOTAL FAT: 8G; SATURATED FAT: 0G; TRANS FAT: 0G; CHOLESTEROL: 0MG; SODIUM: 60MG; TOTAL CARBOHYDRATE: 44G; FIBER: 7G; SUGAR: 13G; PROTEIN: 10G

Overnight oatmeal recipes are so easy to make. Make a batch at the beginning of the week and have enough for the entire week—no cooking involved. You can even add the fruit ahead of time to save an extra step in the morning. With endless combinations, you can keep breakfast heart-healthy and exciting for weeks on end.

1 cup old-fashioned rolled oats, divided

1 cup low-fat soy milk, divided

½ teaspoon vanilla extract, divided

1 cup chopped pears (from about
   2 medium pears), divided

2 tablespoons roasted, shelled,
   unsalted pistachios, divided

1 Using two ½-pint (8-ounce) Mason jars, or other containers with lids, fill each with ½ cup of oatmeal.

2 Stir ½ cup soy milk and ¼ teaspoon vanilla into each jar. Cover and refrigerate overnight.

3 To serve, top each jar with ½ cup of pears and 1 table-spoon of pistachios.

Substitution tip Using the basic oat and milk proportions, here are some additional fruit and nut combinations to try (per serving): ½ cup pitted cherries and 1 tablespoon sliced almonds; ½ cup blueberries and 1 tablespoon cashews; ½ cup chopped strawberries and 1 tablespoon pumpkin seeds.

	5 MAIN INGREDIENTS	BUDGET SAVER	DAIRY FREE	LOW SODIUM	ONE POT	

Steel-Cut Oats with Blueberries and Pecans

Serves 4 | Prep time: 5 minutes | Cook time: 25 minutes

➤ **PER SERVING** CALORIES: 274; TOTAL FAT: 8G; SATURATED FAT: 1G; TRANS FAT: 0G; CHOLESTEROL: 3MG; SODIUM: 56MG; TOTAL CARBOHYDRATE: 44G; FIBER: 7G; SUGAR: 14G; PROTEIN: 11G

Rolled oats and steel-cut oats are both whole grains, but because of the way they are cut, steel-cut oats take slightly longer to digest and rank lower on the glycemic index (a measure of how quickly carbohydrate foods affect blood sugar). With a chewy texture, this stove top recipe is easy to make, creamy, filling, full of fiber, and high in antioxidants from sweet and delicious blueberries.

2 cups nonfat milk, or low-fat milk

1 cup water

1 cup steel-cut oats

2 cups fresh blueberries

¼ cup chopped raw, unsalted pecans, or other nut of choice (**see tip**)

1 In a medium pot over high heat, combine the milk, water, and oats. Bring the mixture to a boil. Reduce the heat to low, cover the pot, and simmer for about 10 minutes, stirring occasionally.

2 Add the blueberries and re-cover the pot. Simmer for 10 minutes more.

3 Turn off the heat and let stand on the hot burner for 5 minutes, until the liquid is absorbed.

4 Top each serving with 1 tablespoon of chopped pecans.

Substitution tip Other cholesterol-lowering nuts you may want to try include almonds, hazelnuts, peanuts, pine nuts, pistachios, and walnuts. Make sure the nuts you choose aren't salted or coated with sugar. All nuts are high in calories, so keep an eye on portion size, which should generally be about ¼ cup or 1 ounce.

5 MAIN INGREDIENTS	30 MINUTES OR FEWER	BUDGET SAVER	LOW SODIUM	ONE POT

Creamy Oat Bran with Apricots

Serves 2 | Prep time: 3 minutes | Cook time: 5 minutes

➤ **PER SERVING** CALORIES: 250; TOTAL FAT: 6G; SATURATED FAT: 1G; TRANS FAT: 0G; CHOLESTEROL: 0MG; SODIUM: 123MG; TOTAL CARBOHYDRATE: 41G; FIBER: 8G; SUGAR: 13G; PROTEIN: 14G

This creamy, hot oat bran breakfast is so delicious you may find you prefer the bran cereal to regular old-fashioned rolled oats. Oat bran is the outer husk of the oat grain, which contains the bulk of its dietary fiber. When mixed with water or milk, it becomes creamy like porridge. A bowl of oat bran contains about 50 percent more fiber than old-fashioned rolled oats, with a similar amount of calories. Apricots add a touch of sweetness, antioxidants, potassium, and even more fiber, and soy milk boosts the protein content.

2 cups low-fat soy milk

1 cup oat bran cereal

¼ teaspoon ground cinnamon

4 fresh or unsweetened dried
   apricots, chopped

Sweetener of choice, such as stevia,
   brown sugar, pure maple syrup,
   or honey (optional)

1 In a medium saucepan over medium heat, stir together the soy milk, oat bran, cinnamon, and apricots. Cook for 3 to 5 minutes, stirring frequently, or until the mixture begins to bubble and boil, and then to thicken.

2 Remove from the heat, portion into bowls, drizzle with sweetener (if using), and serve. The mixture will thicken slightly after removing it from the heat.

5 MAIN INGREDIENTS	30 MINUTES OR FEWER	BUDGET SAVER	DAIRY FREE	LOW SODIUM	NUT FREE	ONE POT	

Overnight Slow Cooker Oatmeal

Serves 4 | Prep time: 10 minutes | Cook time: 9 hours

➤ **PER SERVING** CALORIES: 351; TOTAL FAT: 12G; SATURATED FAT: 1G; TRANS FAT: 0G; CHOLESTEROL: 1MG; SODIUM: 16MG; TOTAL CARBOHYDRATE: 58G; FIBER: 11G; SUGAR: 21G; PROTEIN: 11G

This is an easy-to-make, low-cholesterol triple threat featuring three cholesterol-lowering ingredients: oatmeal, almonds, and apples. Make the oatmeal overnight in a slow cooker, and add flavor and crunch with cinnamon, almonds, and apples in the morning.

Nonstick cooking spray

4 cups water

1 cup steel-cut oats

½ cup skim milk

4 teaspoons ground cinnamon, divided

4 apples, washed, sliced,
  and diced, divided

8 tablespoons chopped raw, unsalted
  almonds, or more to taste, divided

1 Lightly coat your slow cooker insert with cooking spray and combine the water, oats, and milk in it. Cover and cook for 8 to 9 hours (overnight) on low heat.

2 In the morning, stir the oatmeal and portion it into 4 bowls. Top each bowl with 1 teaspoon cinnamon, 1 diced apple, and 2 tablespoons chopped almonds.

3 Refrigerate leftover oatmeal without the toppings in an airtight container. To reheat, in a microwave-safe bowl, combine 1 serving of oatmeal with ¼ to ⅓ cup skim milk, stir, and microwave on high power until hot, stirring after 1 minute. Add the toppings and enjoy.

BUDGET SAVER	LOW SODIUM	ONE POT

Cherry-Coconut Muesli

Prep time: 10 minutes

➤ **PER SERVING** CALORIES: 293; TOTAL FAT: 10G; SATURATED FAT: 3G; TRANS FAT: 0G; CHOLESTEROL: 0MG; SODIUM: 6MG; TOTAL CARBOHYDRATE: 43G; FIBER: 7G; SUGAR: 7G; PROTEIN: 8G

Pronounced muse-lee, this is an uncooked mixture of nuts, seeds, grains, dried fruits, and spices. Muesli can be mixed with nut milks, yogurts, fruit juices, or eaten au natural. So what's the difference between granola and muesli? While they contain similar ingredients, granola contains a fat (oil) and a sweetener, and is baked, whereas muesli doesn't contain any added sugars or oils and is eaten raw or uncooked. Both are delicious, nutrient dense, and easy to make and serve.

2 cups old-fashioned rolled oats

½ cup dried tart cherries

¼ cup coarsely chopped raw, unsalted almonds

¼ cup raw, unsalted pumpkin seeds

2 tablespoons unsweetened flaked coconut

1 teaspoon ground cinnamon

1 teaspoon vanilla extract

1 In a medium bowl, stir together the oats, cherries, almonds, pumpkin seeds, coconut, cinnamon, and vanilla until each ingredient is distributed in the mix. Store in an airtight container, Mason jars, or resealable plastic bags at room temperature.

2 Serve with milk, cold or warm, with fresh fruit and/or yogurt.

Substitution tip Some other ideas for grains, fruits, nuts, and seeds include chia seeds, dried apricots, walnuts, raisins, hemp seeds, sunflower seeds, flaxseed, rye flakes, quinoa flakes, wheat flakes.

	30 MINUTES OR FEWER	BUDGET SAVER	DAIRY FREE	LOW SODIUM	ONE POT	

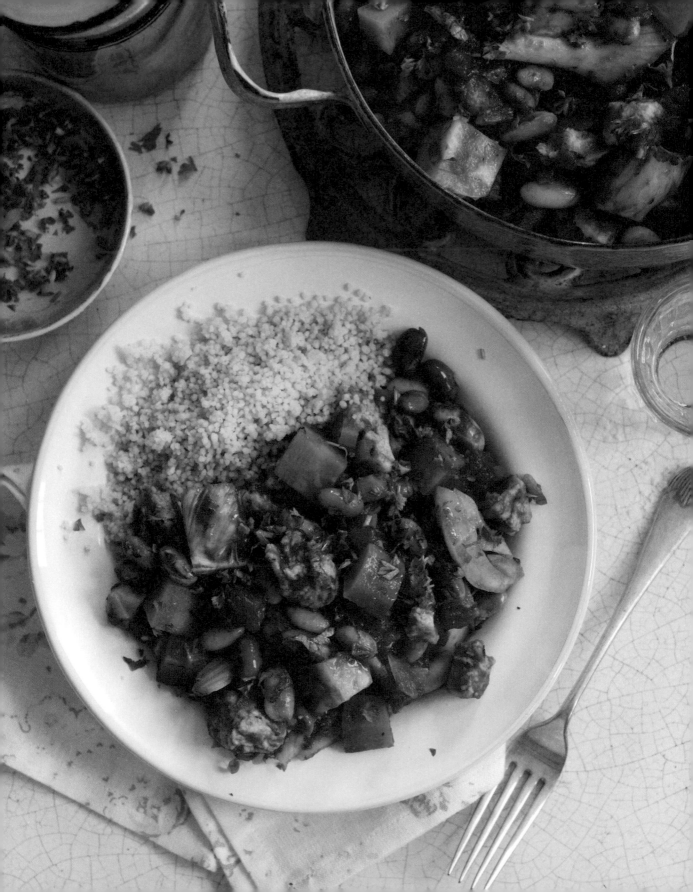

CHAPTER 5

Vegetarian and Vegan Mains

Roasted Veggie and Black Bean Rice Bowl

Serves 4 | Prep time: 10 minutes | Cook time: 30 minutes

➤ **PER SERVING** CALORIES: 207; TOTAL FAT: 4G; SATURATED FAT: 1G; TRANS FAT: 0G; CHOLESTEROL: 0MG; SODIUM: 14MG; TOTAL CARBOHYDRATE: 35G; FIBER: 7G; SUGAR: 2G; PROTEIN: 9G

The blank canvas of brown rice and black beans balances beautifully with the explosive, spicy flavors of the roasted veggies in this incredibly flavorful, cholesterol-lowering rice bowl. Beans are one of the most nutritious foods you can include in your heart-healthy diet, as they are high in soluble fiber, plant protein, B vitamins, and minerals. Simple to prepare, add a touch of avocado, lime, or salsa to this bowl to make it your own.

Nonstick cooking spray

1 tablespoon olive oil

4 garlic cloves, minced

1 teaspoon ground cumin

1 teaspoon chili powder

Freshly ground black pepper

1 medium red onion, diced

1 red bell pepper, diced

1 cup Brussels sprouts, halved

2 cups cooked brown rice, warm

1 (15-ounce) can black beans, drained and rinsed

Lime wedges, for serving (optional)

Avocado slices, for serving (optional)

Fresh cilantro for serving (optional)

1 Preheat the oven to 400°F.

2 Spray a baking sheet with cooking spray and set aside.

3 In a medium bowl, stir together the olive oil, garlic, cumin, chili powder, and pepper until combined.

4 Add the red onion, red bell pepper, and Brussels sprouts and toss to coat. Spread the veggies on the prepared sheet in one layer. Roast for 20 to 30 minutes, stirring occasionally, until the veggies are tender and begin to brown and caramelize.

5 To assemble the bowls, spoon brown rice into 4 bowls, and top with black beans and roasted veggies.

6 Serve with lime wedges, avocado slices, and cilantro (if using).

Did you know? If you usually eat white rice, make it a goal to transition to brown. Brown rice's high magnesium content is good for your heart, its abundant phytonutrient content may protect against various diseases, and its fiber content has been shown to lower cholesterol.

	DAIRY FREE	LOW SODIUM	NUT FREE	ONE POT	

Cheesy Pumpkin Quesadillas

Serves 4 | Prep time: 5 minutes | Cook time: 12 minutes

➤ **PER SERVING** CALORIES: 419; TOTAL FAT: 20G; SATURATED FAT: 4G; TRANS FAT: 0G; CHOLESTEROL: 15MG; SODIUM: 835MG; TOTAL CARBOHYDRATE: 47G; FIBER: 12G; SUGAR: 4G; PROTEIN: 20G

The bright orange color of pumpkin is a dead giveaway that it is loaded with an important antioxidant—beta-carotene—which offers protection against chronic diseases, such as heart disease. An overlooked source of dietary fiber, a one-cup serving has 3 grams, which can keep you feeling fuller longer and keep cholesterol levels in check. Not just for Thanksgiving, this delicious and quick-to-prepare pumpkin quesadilla is also high in potassium for healthy blood pressure.

2 cups canned 100% pure pumpkin
   (not pie filling)
1 teaspoon ground cumin
8 (8-inch) whole-wheat tortillas
4 ounces shredded part-skim
   mozzarella cheese, divided
¼ cup chopped raw, unsalted
   walnuts, divided
½ cup chopped fresh cilantro,
   divided (optional)
2 tablespoons olive oil, divided

1 In a medium bowl, stir together the pumpkin and cumin. Spread the pumpkin over 4 tortillas.

2 Sprinkle each with 1 ounce of mozzarella cheese, 1 tablespoon of walnuts, and 2 tablespoons of cilantro (if using). Top with the remaining 4 tortillas.

3 In a large skillet over medium-high heat, heat 1½ teaspoons of olive oil.

4 Cook the quesadillas, one at a time, for about 3 minutes, turning once and adding more olive oil between batches, until browned. Cut into wedges to serve.

Substitution tip For a different twist, substitute low-sodium, low-fat cottage cheese or ricotta cheese for the mozzarella. Make this vegan by substituting crumbled tofu or vegan cheese.

	5 MAIN INGREDIENTS	30 MINUTES OR FEWER	BUDGET SAVER	ONE POT	

Portobello Baked Eggs with Spinach and Mozzarella

Serves 4 | Prep time: 10 minutes | Cook time: 20 minutes

➤ **PER SERVING** CALORIES: 158; TOTAL FAT: 7G; SATURATED FAT: 3G; TRANS FAT: 0G; CHOLESTEROL: 194MG; SODIUM: 175MG; TOTAL CARBOHYDRATE: 9G; FIBER: 3G; SUGAR: 4G; PROTEIN: 15G

Following a heart-healthy, cholesterol-lowering diet means you need to be moderate with your meat consumption, but it doesn't mean your diet has to be bland. This easy and nutritious recipe uses "meaty" portobello mushroom caps and stuffs them with fiber- and nutrient-rich spinach and protein-packed eggs. With their rich flavor and meaty texture, portobello mushrooms may become your new favorite vegetable.

4 large portobello mushrooms

Olive oil, for cooking

1 cup fresh spinach, washed, dried, and cut into strips, or fresh baby spinach

2 garlic cloves, minced

½ cup shredded part-skim mozzarella cheese

Basil, rosemary, or parsley sprigs, chopped (optional)

4 large eggs

Salt

Freshly ground black pepper

1 Preheat the oven to 425°F.

2 Line a baking sheet with aluminum foil.

3 Wipe the mushroom caps gently with a damp paper towel to remove any dirt. Remove the stems and use a spoon to scrape out the gills. Brush both sides of the mushrooms with a light coating of olive oil, and place them top-side down on the prepared sheet. Bake for 5 minutes.

4 While the mushroom caps bake, heat a large nonstick skillet or sauté pan over medium-high heat and sauté the spinach and garlic in a bit of olive oil for 1 to 2 minutes until the spinach wilts.

	5 MAIN INGREDIENTS	30 MINUTES OR FEWER	LOW SODIUM	NUT FREE	

5 Remove the mushroom caps from the oven and pour out the liquid. Return the mushrooms to the baking sheet, and layer the sautéed spinach, mozzarella cheese, and herbs (if using) into the caps, leaving a "bowl" in the center for the egg.

6 Gently crack one egg into the center of each mushroom cap, on top of the spinach and cheese, and season with salt and pepper. Bake for 8 to 10 minutes, or until the egg whites begin to firm up and the yolks are cooked to your liking.

Did you know? Portobello mushrooms are very low in calories, about 33 for an average cap. One cup of chopped mushrooms has approximately 5 grams of protein and 3 grams of dietary fiber. Made up of about 60 percent water, portobello mushrooms are also a good source of heart-healthy potassium.

Mixed Greens with Lentils and Sliced Apple

Serves 4 | Prep time: 10 minutes | Cook time: 20 minutes

➤ **PER SERVING** CALORIES: 230; TOTAL FAT: 5G; SATURATED FAT: 1G; TRANS FAT: 0G; CHOLESTEROL: 0MG; SODIUM: 55MG; TOTAL CARBOHYDRATE: 49G; FIBER: 17G; SUGAR: 21G; PROTEIN: 11G

This protein- and fiber-rich salad of lentils and apple is a satisfying, cholesterol-lowering vegetarian entrée that's quick to prepare for lunch or a light dinner. While lentils cook very quickly, if you want to save time, swap in drained canned lentils—look for low-sodium choices and rinse them thoroughly before adding to the salad.

1 cup dried green or brown lentils

2 cups water

2 garlic cloves, minced

Pinch salt

6 cups mixed baby greens

4 apples, cored and sliced, divided

4 teaspoons olive oil, divided

¼ cup red wine vinegar, divided

1 Put the lentils into a strainer or colander. Pick them over and remove any shriveled lentils, debris, or rocks. Thoroughly rinse the lentils under running water and transfer to a saucepan.

2 Add the water, garlic, and salt. Bring to a rapid simmer over medium-high heat. Reduce the heat to maintain a very gentle simmer. Cook uncovered for 15 to 20 minutes. You want the lentils to retain some of their shape for use in the salad.

3 Drain the lentils.

4 Divide the baby greens among 4 serving plates. To each plate of greens add one-fourth of the lentils, 1 sliced apple, 1 teaspoon of olive oil, and 1 tablespoon of red wine vinegar. Enjoy.

Did you know? Lentils are marketed in four categories: brown, green, red/yellow, and specialty (e.g., beluga, French). In general, brown and green varieties retain their shape well and are best for salads. Red and yellow tend to disintegrate and are best for soups or in recipes where they will be puréed. Beluga or French green lentils are perfect in salads or featured with pasta, rice, or sautéed vegetables

	30 MINUTES OR FEWER	BUDGET SAVER	DAIRY FREE	LOW SODIUM	NUT FREE	

Vegetarian Cassoulet with Couscous

Serves 4 | Prep time: 10 minutes | Cook time: 40 minutes

➤ **PER SERVING** CALORIES: 489; TOTAL FAT: 8G; SATURATED FAT: 1G; TRANS FAT: 0G; CHOLESTEROL: 0MG; SODIUM: 290MG; TOTAL CARBOHYDRATE: 87G; FIBER: 13G; SUGAR: 9G; PROTEIN: 19G

This vegetarian cassoulet is packed with flavor, plant-based protein, and cholesterol-lowering fiber. Colorful and high in vitamins, minerals, and antioxidants, this filling stew is served with couscous, a quick-cooking high-fiber grain rich in B vitamins.

2 tablespoons olive oil

2 medium sweet potatoes, peeled and diced

1 medium turnip, peeled and chopped

2 teaspoons ground cumin

½ teaspoon ground cinnamon

4 garlic cloves, minced

1 (15-ounce) can kidney beans, drained and rinsed

1 (15-ounce) can pinto beans, drained and rinsed

1 (15-ounce) can diced no-salt-added tomatoes

1 cup low-sodium vegetable broth

Salt

Freshly ground black pepper

1 cup couscous

¼ cup fresh parsley leaves

1 In a large lidded pot over medium-low heat, heat the olive oil.

2 Add the sweet potatoes and turnip. Gently sauté for 10 minutes with the lid loosely on, stirring occasionally.

3 Stir in the cumin, cinnamon, and garlic. Cook for 2 to 3 minutes more.

4 Add the kidney and pinto beans, tomatoes, and vegetable broth. Increase the heat to high and bring the mixture to a boil. Reduce the heat to a gentle simmer. Cover the pot and cook for 20 to 30 minutes. Season with salt and pepper.

5 When the stew is almost finished cooking, prepare the couscous: In a medium pot over high heat, bring 1½ cups water to a boil. Add the couscous, stir once, cover the pot, and remove it from the heat. Let stand 5 minutes and fluff with a fork.

6 Serve the couscous with the cassoulet garnished with fresh parsley.

DAIRY FREE	LOW SODIUM	NUT FREE

Roasted Chickpea–Stuffed Sweet Potatoes with Creamy Tahini Sauce

Serves 4 | Prep time: 10 minutes | Cook time: 40 minutes

➤ **PER SERVING** CALORIES: 371; TOTAL FAT: 17G; SATURATED FAT: 2G; TRANS FAT: 0G; CHOLESTEROL: 0MG; SODIUM: 48MG; TOTAL CARBOHYDRATE: 46G; FIBER: 10G; SUGAR: 23G; PROTEIN: 11G

Simple sweet potatoes make the perfect base for an easy, nourishing meal. A nutritional powerhouse, sweet potatoes are loaded with vitamin A, fiber, potassium, B vitamins, and powerful antioxidants. In this recipe they are loaded up with roasted chickpeas, a high-fiber plant protein, and topped with creamy sesame tahini sauce. Simple, yet big on flavor, you can customize your meal with your favorite toppings.

4 medium sweet potatoes, scrubbed, dried, and pricked all over with a fork

FOR THE OVEN-ROASTED CHICKPEAS

1 (15-ounce) can chickpeas, rinsed, drained, and blotted dry with a paper towel

2 tablespoons olive oil

½ teaspoon ground cumin

Pinch salt

FOR THE CREAMY TAHINI SAUCE

¼ cup tahini

2 garlic cloves, minced

Pinch salt

2 to 3 tablespoons water, as needed

1 Preheat the oven to 400°F.

2 Line two baking sheets with parchment paper or aluminum foil, and place the sweet potatoes on one of the prepared sheets. Bake on the bottom oven rack for about 40 minutes, until the centers of the sweet potatoes are soft when pierced with a knife. Remove from the oven and let cool for a few minutes.

	5 MAIN INGREDIENTS	DAIRY FREE	LOW SODIUM	

TO MAKE THE OVEN-ROASTED CHICKPEAS

Meanwhile, in a medium bowl, stir together the chickpeas, olive oil, cumin, and salt until the chickpeas are evenly coated with the flavorings. Spread them evenly onto the second prepared sheet and roast on the top oven rack for 35 to 40 minutes until crisp and golden, tossing a few times during baking to prevent uneven browning.

TO MAKE THE CREAMY TAHINI SAUCE

In a small bowl, whisk the tahini, garlic, salt, and water as needed until creamy.

TO ASSEMBLE

Slice the potatoes down the center, almost to the bottom but not all the way through. Stuff each sweet potato with the roasted chickpeas and top with the creamy tahini sauce. Serve immediately.

Ingredient tip You can also add your favorite fresh chopped herbs to the oven-roasted chickpeas for additional flavor and nutrients. Parsley and basil both work well. You can also add some vegetables to roast along with the chickpeas, such as a red pepper, Brussels sprouts, red onion, carrots, or asparagus.

Tofu and Vegetable Burritos

Serves 4 | Prep time: 5 minutes, plus 20 to 30 minutes to drain | Cook time: 10 minutes

➤ PER SERVING CALORIES: 304; TOTAL FAT: 16G; SATURATED FAT: 2G; TRANS FAT: 0G; CHOLESTEROL: 0MG; SODIUM: 366MG; TOTAL CARBOHYDRATE: 28G; FIBER: 6G; SUGAR: 2G; PROTEIN: 19G

If you are looking for a simple and healthy recipe for burritos to make at home, this recipe should fit the bill. Completely dairy-free and full of fiber, plant protein, and antioxidant-rich veggies, these burritos will fill you up while adding cholesterol-lowering nutrients to your diet. Once you get the basic recipe down, get creative by switching up the veggies and spices based on your preference.

4 (8-inch) whole-wheat flour tortillas

2 tablespoons olive oil, divided

1 cup diced onion

1 pound extra-firm tofu, drained and pressed dry, chopped into 1-inch cubes (see tip)

2 cups chopped broccoli florets

1 teaspoon ground cumin

Salt

Freshly ground black pepper

Chopped tomato, for topping (optional)

Shredded lettuce, for topping (optional)

Salsa, for topping (optional)

Chopped avocado, for topping (optional)

Fresh cilantro, for topping (optional)

1 In a large dry (no oil used) skillet over medium heat, warm the tortillas for about 30 seconds on each side. Remove and keep warm until needed.

2 Return the skillet to the heat, increase the heat to medium-high, and heat 1 tablespoon of olive oil.

3 Add the onion. Sauté for 1 minute.

4 Add the remaining tablespoon of olive oil, along with the tofu and broccoli. Cook for 4 to 6 minutes, stirring frequently, or until the broccoli is soft and cooked. Remove the pan from the heat.

5 Stir in in the cumin and season with salt and pepper.

6 Place ⅓ to ½ cup of the tofu-vegetable mixture in each flour tortilla. Top with your favorite toppings (if using) and wrap up the burritos. Serve hot.

Ingredient tip Draining your tofu before cooking removes much of the water, giving it a firmer texture. Simply cut the tofu into cubes and place them on a clean dishtowel. Place another dishtowel on top and set something heavy on top, like a cutting board or bowl. Let the dishtowels soak up the moisture for 20 to 30 minutes.

	DAIRY FREE	LOW SODIUM	NUT FREE	

Beet and Bean Burgers

Serves 6 | Prep time: 10 minutes | Cook time: 30 minutes

➤ **PER SERVING** CALORIES: 129; TOTAL FAT: 2G; SATURATED FAT: 0G; TRANS FAT: 0G; CHOLESTEROL: 0MG; SODIUM: 162MG; TOTAL CARBOHYDRATE: 23G; FIBER: 5G; SUGAR: 5G; PROTEIN: 6G

These "meaty" burgers are made from fiber- and protein-rich black beans and heart-healthy beets and oats; they make a perfect replacement for meat on your plate. You'll feel completely satisfied after eating this scrumptious burger, served on a toasty bun piled high with greens. Make a big batch and freeze them for any day you are pressed for time, or when you get that "burger" craving.

1 (15-ounce) can black beans, drained and rinsed

2 cups peeled beet chunks (small chunks)

½ cup oat flour, plus more as needed

2 garlic cloves, minced

2 teaspoons olive oil

½ teaspoon freshly ground black pepper

1 teaspoon ground cumin

2 teaspoons Dijon mustard (optional)

1 teaspoon paprika (optional)

1 Preheat the oven to 375°F.

2 Line a baking sheet with parchment paper and set aside.

3 In a food processor or blender, combine the black beans and beets. Process until combined into a smooth paste. Transfer the mixture to a medium bowl.

4 Add the oat flour, garlic, olive oil, pepper, and cumin, and Dijon mustard and paprika (if using). Stir until well combined. You should be able to handle the mixture and form it into patties. If the mixture is too runny, add 1 tablespoon of oat flour at a time until the desired texture is reached. Using clean hands, form the bean-beet mixture into 8 patties. Place them on the prepared sheet and bake for 25 to 30 minutes until the edges are crispy, flipping halfway through the baking time.

5 Serve with your favorite burger toppings.

Did you know? Beets are rich in nitrates that the body converts to nitric oxide, a compound that relaxes and dilates blood vessels, which translates into better circulation and lower blood pressure. They are also a rich source of insoluble fiber and numerous minerals, vitamins, and phytonutrients.

5 MAIN INGREDIENTS	BUDGET SAVER	DAIRY FREE	LOW SODIUM	NUT FREE

Herbed Chickpeas

Serves 4 | Prep time: 10 minutes | Cook time: 15 minutes

➤ **PER SERVING** CALORIES: 350; TOTAL FAT: 14G; SATURATED FAT: 2G; TRANS FAT: 0G; CHOLESTEROL: 0MG; SODIUM: 73MG; TOTAL CARBOHYDRATE: 46G; FIBER: 13G; SUGAR: 11G; PROTEIN: 13G

Rich in both fiber and protein, this vegan main dish is crispy, creamy, and simple to prepare. Chickpeas are high in cholesterol-lowering fiber, and carrots, garlic, and onion add valuable inflammation-reducing antioxidants. With just five main ingredients, these chickpeas should become a staple in your kitchen. Serve as a main entrée or pair with eggs, cooked grains, grilled meats, or a fresh green salad.

2 (15-ounce) cans chickpeas, drained and rinsed

4 garlic cloves, crushed

2 cups grated carrot

1 cup diced red onion

3 tablespoons olive oil

Salt

Freshly ground black pepper

3 cups chopped mixed herbs such as parsley, cilantro, chives, and basil

1 In a large skillet or Dutch oven over medium heat, combine the chickpeas, garlic, carrot, red onion, and olive oil. Season with salt and pepper. Cook for 10 to 15 minutes, stirring occasionally, until the chickpeas are crisped and some have split open.

2 Remove from the heat, stir in the herbs, and serve warm.

Did you know? Adding a little spice to your diet is a delectable way to edge cholesterol levels downward. Many herbs and spices are high in antioxidant and anti-inflammatory activity, especially garlic, onion, ginger, and turmeric. One teaspoon of freshly grated ginger would work well in this recipe with fresh parsley and chives.

5 MAIN INGREDIENTS	30 MINUTES OR FEWER	BUDGET SAVER	DAIRY FREE	LOW SODIUM	NUT FREE	ONE POT	

Stuffed Zucchini Boats

Serves 4 | Prep time: 10 minutes | Cook time: 35 minutes

➤ **PER SERVING** CALORIES: 142; TOTAL FAT: 8G; SATURATED FAT: 1G; TRANS FAT: 0G; CHOLESTEROL: 0MG; SODIUM: 51MG; TOTAL CARBOHYDRATE: 17G; FIBER: 5G; SUGAR: 7G; PROTEIN: 4G

These vegan stuffed zucchini are a delicious and hearty meatless Monday meal option, or the perfect side to grilled or roasted tofu, poultry, or fish. This recipe uses the squash as a boat for a simple sautéed mix of onion, eggplant, and bell peppers. It's a delicious, plant-based way to achieve a meaty texture in a satisfying light dish.

2 tablespoons olive oil, divided

1 white onion, chopped

1 large bell pepper, any color, chopped

1 small eggplant, chopped
   (about 4 cups)

1 cup frozen green peas, thawed

2 zucchini, halved lengthwise,
   flesh scooped out and reserved,
   leaving a ½-inch shell

Salt

Freshly ground black pepper

1 Preheat the oven to 400°F.

2 In a large nonstick skillet over medium-high heat, heat 1½ teaspoons of olive oil.

3 Add the onion, bell pepper, and eggplant. Sauté for about 5 minutes until tender.

4 Add the peas and reserved zucchini flesh and continue cooking for 2 minutes more. Season with salt and pepper.

5 Drizzle the bottom of a baking dish with 1½ teaspoons of olive oil, and place the zucchini halves in the dish, skin-side down.

6 Fill the zucchini boats equally with the veggie mixture. Drizzle the remaining tablespoon of olive oil over the tops. Bake for 20 to 25 minutes, until the zucchini are tender.

Substitution tip To boost the protein content of this recipe, swap the peas for lentils or black beans. You could also sprinkle the zucchini boats with your favorite low-fat cheese.

	5 MAIN INGREDIENTS	BUDGET SAVER	DAIRY FREE	LOW SODIUM	NUT FREE	

Fried Cauliflower Rice

Serves 4 | Prep time: 5 minutes | Cook time: 15 minutes

➤ **PER SERVING** CALORIES: 136; TOTAL FAT: 5G; SATURATED FAT: 1G; TRANS FAT: 0G; CHOLESTEROL: 47MG; SODIUM: 270MG; TOTAL CARBOHYDRATE: 16G; FIBER: 6G; SUGAR: 6G; PROTEIN: 9G

Traditional fried rice tastes terrific, but it is also high in refined carbohydrates, fat, calories, and sodium. Thankfully, cauliflower is a great substitute for rice when you are looking for something healthier, lower in carbs, grain-free, high-fiber, and protein-rich. Bonus: You can have this delicious main dish that everyone will love on the table in 20 minutes.

1 medium (about 24-ounce) head
    cauliflower, rinsed, cored, and
    coarsely chopped into florets

2 large egg whites

1 large egg

Nonstick cooking spray,
    or olive oil mister

1 tablespoon sesame oil

6 scallions, diced, whites and
    greens separated

1 cup frozen peas

4 garlic cloves, minced

1 tablespoon low-sodium
    soy sauce, or to taste

1 Place half the cauliflower florets in a food processor and pulse until the cauliflower has the texture of rice—don't over process or it will become mushy. Transfer to a medium bowl, set aside, and repeat with the remaining cauliflower.

2 In a small bowl, combine the egg whites and egg. Beat together with a fork.

3 Heat a large skillet, sauté pan, or wok over medium heat. Spray the pan with cooking spray or your olive oil mister.

4 Add the eggs and scramble for 1 to 2 minutes, stirring a few times, until set. Transfer to a small bowl and set aside.

30 MINUTES OR FEWER	BUDGET SAVER	DAIRY FREE	LOW SODIUM	NUT FREE

5 Return the skillet to the heat, increase the heat to medium-high, and add the sesame oil, scallion whites, peas, and garlic. Sauté for 3 to 4 minutes until soft.

6 Add the cauliflower rice to the pan along with the soy sauce. Stir to mix, cover the pan, and cook for 5 to 6 minutes, stirring frequently, until the cauliflower is slightly crispy on the outside, but tender on the inside.

7 Stir in the eggs, remove the pan from the heat, and top with the scallion greens. Serve hot.

Ingredient tip You can save time by purchasing already "riced" cauliflower. Find it in the produce section of most grocery stores and big-box retailers like Walmart.

Slow Cooker White Beans and Barley

Serves 4 | Prep time: 10 minutes | Cook time: 8 hours on low heat or 4 hours on high heat

➤ **PER SERVING** CALORIES: 371; TOTAL FAT: 5G; SATURATED FAT: 1G; TRANS FAT: 0G; CHOLESTEROL: 0MG; SODIUM: 222MG; TOTAL CARBOHYDRATE: 71G; FIBER: 16G; SUGAR: 9G; PROTEIN: 14G

Incorporating more hulled barley into your cholesterol-lowering diet is definitely worth the time investment for the returns on your health. To make things easier, a slow cooker is used to prepare this fiber- and protein-rich soup loaded with immunity boosters. Set this to cooking on a Sunday morning and enjoy a hearty nutrient-rich stew for dinner.

1 tablespoon olive oil

1 cup chopped onion

Salt

Freshly ground black pepper

4 cups low-sodium vegetable broth

1 (15-ounce) can white beans, drained and rinsed

1 (14.5-ounce) can crushed no-salt-added tomatoes

1 cup chopped carrot

1 cup hulled barley

1 (10-ounce) package frozen spinach

2 teaspoons dried rosemary

1 In a large nonstick skillet over medium-high heat, heat the olive oil.

2 Add the onion. Cook for about 5 minutes, stirring frequently, until softened. Season with salt and pepper. Transfer the onion to a 5- or 6-quart slow cooker.

3 Add the vegetable broth, white beans, tomatoes, carrot, barley, spinach, and rosemary. Stir to combine. Cover the cooker and cook for 4 hours on high heat or for 8 hours on low heat, until the carrots are tender. Serve hot.

	BUDGET SAVER	DAIRY FREE	LOW SODIUM	NUT FREE	

Lentil and Spinach Stew

Serves 4 | Prep time: 5 minutes | Cook time: 40 minutes

➤ **PER SERVING** CALORIES: 233; TOTAL FAT: 7G; SATURATED FAT: 1G; TRANS FAT: 0G; CHOLESTEROL: 0MG; SODIUM: 90MG; TOTAL CARBOHYDRATE: 39G; FIBER: 19G; SUGAR: 8G; PROTEIN: 19G

Lentil soup is one of those quintessential comfort foods that's full of flavor—and it's exceedingly nutritious. One cup of lentils contains 63 percent of our recommended dietary fiber along with ample protein, iron, potassium, and other important vitamins and minerals. This recipe includes meaty portobello mushrooms to create a perfect bowl of stew that satisfies to the core.

6 cups water, divided

1 cup green lentils, rinsed

2 tablespoons olive oil

3 garlic cloves, minced

3 medium portobello mushrooms, thickly sliced

1 (6-ounce) can no-salt-added tomato paste

1 (10-ounce) package frozen spinach

Salt

Freshly ground black pepper

1 In a large, lidded pot over high heat, combine 4 cups of water and the lentils. Bring to a boil and cook for 10 minutes while you prepare the rest of the ingredients.

2 In a large skillet or sauté pan over medium heat, combine the olive oil, garlic, and mushrooms. Gently sauté for 5 to 8 minutes, until browned and softened.

3 Reduce the heat under the lentils to medium-low and stir in the tomato paste, the remaining 2 cups of water, the spinach, and the mushrooms and garlic. Simmer for 15 minutes, stirring occasionally.

4 Season with salt and pepper. Cover the pot, reduce the heat to low, and let the flavors mingle for 5 to 10 minutes, stirring occasionally. Serve hot.

Substitution tip Other vegetables you may want to add to your stew are chopped onion, sliced carrots, or sliced celery. You can also add your favorite spices, such as 1 teaspoon dried thyme, basil, or tarragon.

	5 MAIN INGREDIENTS	BUDGET SAVER	DAIRY FREE	LOW SODIUM	NUT FREE	

Garlicky Black Bean Soup

Serves 4 | Prep time: 5 minutes | Cook time: 15 minutes

➤ **PER SERVING** CALORIES: 215; TOTAL FAT: 0G; SATURATED FAT: 0G; TRANS FAT: 0G; CHOLESTEROL: 0MG; SODIUM: 31MG; TOTAL CARBOHYDRATE: 40G; FIBER: 11G; SUGAR: 8G; PROTEIN: 12G

With an excellent nutritional profile, beans are a significant source of protein, fiber, and iron, plus they are extremely affordable. While this recipe may look simplistic, it delivers on taste and nutrition. And it's easy to customize, just use your favorite seasonings and toppings.

2 (15-ounce) cans black beans,
    drained and rinsed, divided
1 (14-ounce) can no-salt-added,
    fire-roasted diced tomatoes
1 cup water
4 garlic cloves, minced
1 teaspoon ground cumin
½ cup fresh cilantro, chopped
Diced avocado, for topping (optional)

1 In a large pot over high heat, stir together 1 can of black beans, the tomatoes, water, garlic, and cumin. Bring to a boil. Cook for 10 minutes, stirring occasionally.

2 Using an immersion blender (or in a regular blender, working in batches if necessary), blend the soup until thickened.

3 Return the soup to the pot, stir in the remaining can of black beans, and cook for 5 minutes more. Serve warm garnished with cilantro and avocado (if using).

Did you know? The United Nations chose 2016 as the International Year of the Pulses. Examples of pulses include dry peas, lentils, beans, and chickpeas. They were chosen because they are drought-resistant, have a great nutritional profile, and are a sustainable and environmentally friendly crop option. Consider committing to reduce your carbon footprint and eat pulses at least once a week.

5 MAIN INGREDIENTS	30 MINUTES OR FEWER	BUDGET SAVER	DAIRY FREE	LOW SODIUM	NUT FREE	ONE POT

Veggie Chili

Serves 4 | Prep time: 5 minutes | Cook time: 10 minutes

➤ **PER SERVING** CALORIES: 275; TOTAL FAT: 1G; SATURATED FAT: 0G; TRANS FAT: 0G; CHOLESTEROL: 0MG; SODIUM: 87MG; TOTAL CARBOHYDRATE: 54G; FIBER: 12G; SUGAR: 11G; PROTEIN: 14G

A tried and true, quick-to-prepare healthy chili recipe is an essential item in every cook's arsenal. Making your own chili is much more nutritious and lower in sodium than premade chili, plus it's easy to make using basic pantry ingredients and whatever spices you have on hand. High in fiber and protein, you could double this recipe for freezing.

1 (14-ounce) can no-salt-added, fire-roasted chopped tomatoes

1 cup low-sodium vegetable broth

2 (15-ounce) cans pinto beans (or your favorite bean), drained and rinsed

1 (15-ounce) can corn, drained and rinsed

1 tablespoon chili powder

1 In a large pot over high heat, stir together the tomatoes, vegetable broth, pinto beans, corn, and chili powder. Bring to a boil, reduce the heat to low, and simmer for 8 to 10 minutes.

2 Serve hot topped with your favorite chili garnishes.

Ingredient tip Canned beans are a convenient, economical, and healthy addition to a cholesterol-lowering diet. Stock your pantry with a variety so you have them on hand for preparing meals in a flash. Just remember to drain the beans in a colander and rinse them thoroughly with cold water to remove the sodium and preservatives.

Preparation tip If you like, add a 10-ounce package of frozen spinach or a diced bell pepper, or other vegetables as desired.

5 MAIN INGREDIENTS	30 MINUTES OR FEWER	BUDGET SAVER	DAIRY FREE	LOW SODIUM	NUT FREE	ONE POT

Avocado Pesto Brown Rice

Serves 4 | Prep time: 5 minutes | Cook time: 45 minutes

➤ **PER SERVING**   CALORIES: 346; TOTAL FAT: 21G; SATURATED FAT: 2G; TRANS FAT: 0G; CHOLESTEROL: 0MG;
SODIUM: 4MG; TOTAL CARBOHYDRATE: 38G; FIBER: 5G; SUGAR: 1G; PROTEIN: 5G

This super simple, healthy, and flavorful avocado pesto brown rice is high in filling fiber and heart-healthy monounsaturated fats. Brown basmati rice is a very long-grained and aromatic rice with a nutty flavor and distinctive texture. Many people are nervous about cooking whole-grain rice, but it is actually quite simple, and this variety cooks up in about 40 minutes. With a bright green flavor, this creamy dish is perfect for an easy weeknight dinner.

1 cup brown basmati rice

2¼ cups water, divided,
   plus more as needed

1 large avocado, peeled, pitted,
   and coarsely chopped

1 cup packed fresh basil leaves

¼ cup pine nuts

Juice of 1 lemon

2 tablespoons olive oil

Salt

Freshly ground black pepper

1 In a medium saucepan over medium heat, combine the rice and 2 cups of water. Bring to a boil. Reduce the heat to a gentle simmer, stir, cover the saucepan, and cook for 30 to 40 minutes until the water is completely absorbed. Remove from the heat and let stand, covered, for 5 minutes. Alternatively, use a rice cooker.

2 Meanwhile, in a blender or food processor, combine the avocado, basil, pine nuts, lemon juice, olive oil, and the remaining ¼ cup of water. Purée the mixture until smooth. Season with salt and pepper, and add more water if needed, puréeing until the mixture is the consistency of sour cream.

3 Fluff the rice with a fork and gently fold the green dressing into the warm rice. Serve immediately.

5 MAIN INGREDIENTS	DAIRY FREE	LOW SODIUM

Eggplant and Chickpea Curry

Serves 4 | Prep time: 10 minutes | Cook time: 30 minutes

➤ **PER SERVING** CALORIES: 209; TOTAL FAT: 6G; SATURATED FAT: 1G; TRANS FAT: 0G; CHOLESTEROL: 0MG; SODIUM: 22MG; TOTAL CARBOHYDRATE: 35G; FIBER: 11G; SUGAR: 9G; PROTEIN: 9G

Eggplant shines in this simple, yet flavorful dish. Great for those new to curries, this foolproof recipe couldn't be easier. Make a big pot on a Sunday night and enjoy leftovers for lunch during the week. Full of fiber and plant protein, this antioxidant-rich dish can be enjoyed over rice or quinoa, or rolled into a whole-wheat wrap for a curry burrito.

1 tablespoon olive oil

1 onion, chopped

2 pints cherry tomatoes, halved

1 eggplant (about 1 pound),
 cut into ½-inch pieces

2 teaspoons curry powder

Pinch salt

¼ teaspoon freshly ground
 black pepper

1 (15-ounce) can chickpeas,
 drained and rinsed

½ cup fresh basil leaves (optional)

¼ cup plain low-fat Greek yogurt
 (optional)

1 In a medium saucepan over medium-high heat, heat the olive oil.

2 Add the onion. Cook for 4 to 6 minutes, stirring occasionally, until softened.

3 Stir in the tomatoes, eggplant, curry powder, salt, and pepper. Cook for about 2 minutes stirring, until fragrant.

4 Add 2 cups water and bring the mixture to a boil. Reduce heat to low and simmer, partially covered, for 12 to 15 minutes until the eggplant is tender.

5 Stir in the chickpeas and cook for about 3 minutes just until heated through. Remove from the heat and stir in the basil (if using). Serve over your favorite whole grain or in a whole-wheat tortilla. Top with the yogurt (if using).

Ingredient tip Choose firm, heavy eggplants with shiny skins. Keep refrigerated and use within a few days. Eggplant is very low in calories and a very good source of dietary fiber, thiamin, and copper. It is also a good source of heart-healthy potassium and phytonutrients.

5 MAIN INGREDIENTS	DAIRY FREE	LOW SODIUM	NUT FREE	ONE POT

Butternut Squash Mac and Cheese

Serves 4 | Prep time: 5 minutes | Cook time: 20 minutes

➤ **PER SERVING** CALORIES: 398; TOTAL FAT: 10G; SATURATED FAT: 2G; TRANS FAT: 0G; CHOLESTEROL: 5MG; SODIUM: 133MG; TOTAL CARBOHYDRATE: 65G; FIBER: 10G; SUGAR: 6G; PROTEIN: 14G

Macaroni and cheese is a classic American comfort food; however, boxed mac and cheese is full of sodium, preservatives, and unhealthy fats. A few simple substitutions are all you need to create a veggie- and fiber-packed healthy version that the whole family will love. Creamy puréed butternut squash takes the place of some of the cheese while still maintaining the traditional taste and color of this dish. You'll love this guilt-free, creative, and delicious recipe.

8 ounces whole-wheat elbow macaroni

3 cups peeled, seeded (1-inch) butternut squash cubes

1 cup nonfat or low-fat dairy or nondairy milk

Salt

Freshly ground black pepper

2 tablespoons olive oil, divided

¼ cup freshly grated Parmigiano-Reggiano cheese

⅓ cup whole-wheat panko bread crumbs

Fresh parsley leaves, for serving (optional)

Freshly grated nutmeg, for serving (optional)

1 Fill a large pot with water, place it over high heat, and bring to a boil.

2 Add the macaroni and cook until al dente, about 1 minute less than the package instructions. Drain, reserving about ¼ cup of the pasta water.

3 Meanwhile, in a medium saucepan over medium-high heat, combine the butternut squash and milk. Season with salt and pepper. Bring to a simmer. Reduce the heat to low, cover the saucepan, and cook for 8 to 10 minutes until the squash is fork-tender. Transfer to a blender or food processor, working in batches if necessary, and purée until smooth.

	5 MAIN INGREDIENTS	30 MINUTES OR FEWER	LOW SODIUM	NUT FREE	

4 Place a large skillet or sauté pan over medium heat. Add 1 tablespoon of olive oil. Once hot, add the squash purée. Bring to a simmer and cook for about 5 minutes until thickened.

5 Stir in the cheese to combine. Remove from the heat and set aside.

6 In a small skillet or sauté pan over medium heat, add the remaining tablespoon of olive oil.

7 Stir in the bread crumbs and toast for 2 to 3 minutes, stirring occasionally, until golden brown. Remove from the heat and set aside.

8 Add the pasta to the sauce, and some of the pasta water to loosen it. Garnish with the toasted bread crumbs. Serve warm, sprinkled with fresh parsley and nutmeg (if using).

Ingredient tip To boost the fiber and nutrient content of this dish, add 1 to 2 cups cauliflower florets. Cook and purée with the squash.

Pasta with Baby Spinach, Herbs, and Ricotta

Serves 4 | Prep time: 5 minutes | Cook time: 20 minutes

➤ **PER SERVING** CALORIES: 384; TOTAL FAT: 13G; SATURATED FAT: 4G; TRANS FAT: 0G; CHOLESTEROL: 0MG; SODIUM: 284MG; TOTAL CARBOHYDRATE: 50G; FIBER: 7G; SUGAR: 4G; PROTEIN: 19G

This quick and easy dish will satisfy any craving for decadent, creamy pasta. The low-fat ricotta cheese replaces the high-fat cream found in similar creamy white pasta dishes, while the spinach and lemon zest bring a bright freshness to the bowl. The whole-grain pasta adds valuable fiber for heart health and to keep you feeling full.

2 tablespoons olive oil

1 yellow onion, finely chopped

8 ounces fresh baby spinach, chopped

1½ cups low-fat ricotta cheese

Zest of ½ lemon, finely grated

Salt

Freshly ground black pepper

8 ounces whole-grain pasta
   (use your favorite shape)

¼ cup fresh basil leaves (optional)

1 In a large skillet over medium-high heat, heat the olive oil.

2 Add the onion. Cook for 6 to 8 minutes, stirring occasionally, until softened.

3 Add the spinach and cook for about 3 minutes more, stirring until just wilted.

4 Stir in the ricotta and lemon zest, and season with salt and pepper. Keep warm over very low heat.

5 Cook the pasta in a large pot of boiling water according to the package directions until al dente. Set aside 1 cup of the pasta cooking water and drain the pasta well. Add the drained pasta to the skillet and toss to coat, adding some of the pasta water to loosen the sauce as needed. Top with the basil (if using) and serve immediately.

5 MAIN INGREDIENTS	30 MINUTES OR FEWER	LOW SODIUM	NUT FREE

Gemelli Salad with Green Beans and Pistachios

Serves 4 | Prep time: 10 minutes | Cook time: 10 minutes

➤ **PER SERVING** CALORIES: 432; TOTAL FAT: 22G; SATURATED FAT: 3G; TRANS FAT: 0G; CHOLESTEROL: 0MG; SODIUM: 98MG; TOTAL CARBOHYDRATE: 49G; FIBER: 8G; SUGAR: 3G; PROTEIN: 11G

Gemelli is a type of pasta made of short pieces of pasta shaped on the horizontal plane, like the letter "S" then twisted together. This type of pasta lends itself well to salads and soups; however, for the most cholesterol-lowering benefits, choose a whole-grain variety. If whole-wheat pasta doesn't appeal to you, boost the fiber content of this recipe by adding more vegetables or a can of drained and rinsed beans. Used in this recipe with fiber-rich green beans and heart-healthy pistachios, the gemelli is seasoned with fresh thyme and lemon zest for a light and refreshing dish.

8 ounces gemelli

2 cups cut green beans

½ cup shelled, unsalted pistachios

2 tablespoons fresh thyme
    leaves, divided

2 tablespoons grated lemon
    zest, divided

¼ cup olive oil

2 garlic cloves, minced (optional)

2 tablespoons balsamic vinegar
    (optional)

Salt

Freshly ground black pepper

1 In a large pot of boiling water over high heat, cook the pasta according to the package directions. Halfway through the cooking time, add the green beans and finish cooking. Drain and rinse the pasta and beans under cold water, and transfer to a large bowl.

2 Add the pistachios, 1 tablespoon of thyme, and 1 tablespoon of lemon zest. Gently toss to combine.

3 In a small bowl, whisk the remaining 1 tablespoon of thyme, 1 tablespoon of lemon zest, the olive oil, and garlic and vinegar (if using). Season with salt and pepper. Whisk again. Drizzle over the pasta mixture and gently toss to coat. Serve immediately.

	5 MAIN INGREDIENTS	30 MINUTES OR FEWER	BUDGET SAVER	DAIRY FREE	LOW SODIUM	

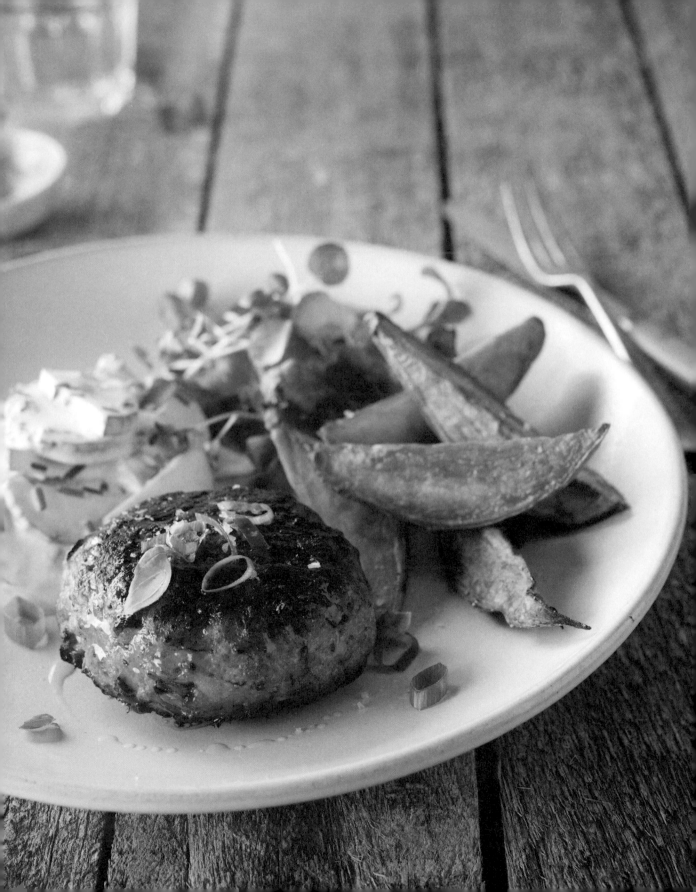

CHAPTER 6

Poultry Mains

Sheet Pan Chicken Fajitas with Fresh Sauce

Serves 4 | Prep time: 10 minutes | Cook time: 25 minutes

➤ **PER SERVING** CALORIES: 234; TOTAL FAT: 6G; SATURATED FAT: 2G; TRANS FAT: 0G; CHOLESTEROL: 65MG; SODIUM: 257MG; TOTAL CARBOHYDRATE: 20G; FIBER: 10G; SUGAR: 3G; PROTEIN: 32G

Restaurant-style Mexican food can often be loaded in calories, unhealthy fats, and sodium. These fajitas prove that Mexican fare can also be super-clean and healthy. Making these fajitas on a sheet pan allows the use of minimal oils, and a freshly prepared spicy sauce cuts down on sodium and preservatives. Choose whole-grain tortillas for your wrap or make an amazing fajita salad by tossing this mixture with the sauce and some shredded lettuce.

FOR THE FAJITAS

1 pound boneless, skinless chicken
    breast, cut into 1-inch slices

2 bell peppers, any color,
    cut into thick slices

Oil olive, for drizzling

4 whole-grain flour or corn
    tortillas, warmed

Diced avocado, for topping (optional)

Low-fat sour cream, for topping
    (optional)

Shredded lettuce, for topping (optional)

FOR THE FRESH SAUCE

1 jalapeño pepper, stemmed
    and seeded

Pinch salt

2 medium tomatoes, stems cut out

½ onion, diced

1 bunch fresh cilantro, minced

TO MAKE THE FAJITAS

1 Preheat the oven to 375°F.

2 Line a rimmed sheet pan with parchment paper and, on it, toss together the chicken and bell peppers with a drizzle of olive oil. Spread the chicken and peppers into an even layer. Bake for 20 to 25 minutes, until the chicken is cooked through and the bell peppers are tender.

3 Remove the chicken and peppers from oven, and divide the mixture among the warmed tortillas. Serve with the fresh sauce and add toppings as desired.

DAIRY FREE	LOW SODIUM	NUT FREE

TO MAKE THE FRESH SAUCE

1 While the chicken and peppers cook, place the jalapeño in a small microwave-safe bowl. Microwave for 2 to 2½ minutes on high power until it is wrinkled, but has not turned black. Remove from the microwave, add the salt, and set aside.

2 Place the tomatoes in a shallow microwave-safe bowl. Microwave on high power for 2 to 3 minutes until soft but not mushy.

3 Remove the jalapeño from bowl, but reserve the water-salt mixture left from cooking. Dice the jalapeño, being very careful of the seeds, and set aside. Do not touch your eyes or face until you have thoroughly washed your hands, or wear food-safe kitchen gloves while handling it. Transfer the diced jalapeño with the water-salt mixture to a food processor or blender. Add the tomatoes without their juices and blend until there are still some tomato chunks remaining. Pour the mixture into a bowl, and stir in the onion and cilantro. Set aside until serving.

Ingredient tip You can also make this recipe by using a rotisserie chicken; however, most retailers heavily brine and season their rotisserie chickens, which means they can be very high in sodium, saturated fat, and cholesterol.

Easy Herb-Baked Chicken Breasts

Serves 2 | Prep time: 10 minutes | Cook time 15 minutes

➤ **PER SERVING** CALORIES: 293; TOTAL FAT: 18G; SATURATED FAT: 4G; TRANS FAT: 0G; CHOLESTEROL: 65MG; SODIUM: 49MG; TOTAL CARBOHYDRATE: 7G; FIBER: 1G; SUGAR: 1G; PROTEIN: 26G

This tasty chicken recipe gets its flavor from fresh herbs and vegetables baked with the chicken. With cholesterol-lowering phytochemicals from the garlic and shallots, this nutritious entrée is satisfying while being low in calories and added fats.

2 (4-ounce) boneless, skinless chicken breasts

Freshly ground black pepper

Salt

2 shallots, minced

4 garlic cloves, minced

1 cup cherry tomatoes, halved

2 tablespoons olive oil

¼ cup torn fresh basil leaves, or 2 thyme sprigs

1 Preheat the oven or a toaster oven to 400°F.

2 Season the chicken breasts on both sides with pepper and just a pinch of salt. Place the chicken in a baking dish.

3 In a medium bowl, stir together the shallots, garlic, and tomatoes. Drizzle with the olive oil and season with pepper. Cover the chicken with the vegetable mixture. Bake for 10 to 15 minutes until an instant-read thermometer registers 165°F.

4 Sprinkle the basil over the chicken and serve immediately.

5 MAIN INGREDIENTS	30 MINUTES OR FEWER	BUDGET SAVER	DAIRY FREE	LOW SODIUM	NUT FREE	

Chicken and Zucchini Burgers

Serves 4 | Prep time: 10 minutes | Cook time: 15 minutes

➤ **PER SERVING** CALORIES: 249; TOTAL FAT: 13G; SATURATED FAT: 4G; TRANS FAT: 0G; CHOLESTEROL: 132MG; SODIUM: 122MG; TOTAL CARBOHYDRATE: 10G; FIBER: 2G; SUGAR: 2G; PROTEIN: 24G

Eating a low-cholesterol diet means exploring creative and healthy new ways to enjoy your favorite foods. These chicken and zucchini burgers are super tasty and, of course, easy to make. The bread crumbs on the outside give them a crunchy coating, while the zucchini keeps them moist and adds valuable fiber, vitamins, and minerals. Eat these in a whole-grain bun, in lettuce leaves, or open face with your favorite toppings. Serve with Baked Sweet Potato Fries (page 159) for a true burger experience.

1 medium zucchini, finely shredded
(see tip)

1 small onion, finely shredded
(see tip)

1 pound lean ground
white meat chicken

1 large egg

½ cup whole-wheat panko
bread crumbs, divided

1 teaspoon freshly ground black pepper

Chopped scallions, white and green
parts, for garnish (optional)

1 Preheat a grill to medium-high heat, or a grill pan over medium-high heat.

2 Squeeze the shredded zucchini in small handfuls to release most of the water.

3 In a large bowl, combine the zucchini, onion, chicken, egg, ¼ cup of the bread crumbs, and the pepper. Using clean hands, mix the ingredients together and form the mixture into 4 patties.

4 Pour the remaining ¼ cup of bread crumbs onto a plate. Coat both sides of each patty in the crumbs.

5 Place the patties on the grill and cook for 6 to 7 minutes. Flip, and grill for 3 to 4 minutes more, or until the internal temperature reaches 160°F. Serve the burgers topped with the scallions (if using) and with your favorite toppings and sides.

Ingredient tip Ground chicken is similar to ground turkey in its appearance and nutrition content. Just like ground turkey, the percentage lean (in ground chicken, usually 80% to 95% lean) depends on the amounts of dark meat and white meat used. To keep saturated fat in check, choose 90% to 95% lean. Onion and zucchini can be shredded using a box grater or plane grater by pushing the vegetables through the large-holes of the grating surface and moving them to the bottom of the grater.

5 MAIN INGREDIENTS	30 MINUTES OR FEWER	DAIRY FREE	LOW SODIUM	NUT FREE

Lemon Chicken with Spinach

Serves 4 | Prep time: 5 minutes | Cook time: 15 minutes

➤ **PER SERVING** CALORIES: 213; TOTAL FAT: 8G; SATURATED FAT: 2G; TRANS FAT: 0G; CHOLESTEROL: 65MG; SODIUM: 301MG; TOTAL CARBOHYDRATE: 8G; FIBER: 3G; SUGAR: 3G; PROTEIN: 28G

This fresh, flavorful, and healthy recipe is cooked in one pan and ready in 20 minutes. Chicken breast is a lean, low-cholesterol, low-calorie source of high-quality protein to keep you feeling full and satisfied. The chunks of juicy chicken are sautéed with garlic, fresh lemon, and basil with vitamin-, mineral-, and fiber-rich spinach to make a complete meal. You can bulk it up further with additional veggies, serve it over brown rice, or toss it on salad greens.

1 tablespoon olive oil

½ large yellow onion, finely chopped (about 1 cup)

4 garlic cloves, minced

1 pound boneless, skinless chicken breast, cut into ¾-inch pieces

1½ tablespoons low-sodium soy sauce

¼ teaspoon freshly ground black pepper, plus more as needed

6 cups loosely packed fresh baby spinach

1 tablespoon lemon zest

2 tablespoons freshly squeezed lemon juice

2 cups fresh basil leaves

Salt

1 In a large skillet over medium heat, heat the olive oil until hot.

2 Add the onion. Cook for about 4 minutes, stirring frequently, until softened.

3 Add the garlic. Cook about 30 seconds, until fragrant.

4 Add the chicken, increase the heat to medium-high, and cook for 3 minutes, browning all sides.

5 Stir in the soy sauce and pepper. Cook for about 3 minutes more, until the chicken is completely cooked through.

6 Stir in the spinach, a few handfuls at a time, letting the heat of the pan wilt it as it cooks.

7 Stir in the lemon zest, lemon juice, and basil. Cook for about 1 minute, stirring, until the basil wilts. Taste, and season with salt and more pepper as desired.

Did you know? Cholesterol-lowering flavonoids are highest in the outer layers of an onion. To retain as many nutrients as possible, peel away only the onion's thin, papery layer and leave its fleshy layers intact. Additionally, it is best to cook onions in a liquid or sauté over low heat, as the antioxidants are transferred into the cooking liquid.

30 MINUTES OR FEWER	DAIRY FREE	LOW SODIUM	NUT FREE	ONE POT

Rosemary Chicken and Vegetables
Sheet Pan Dinner

Serves 4 | Prep time: 10 minutes | Cook time: 30 minutes

➤ **PER SERVING** CALORIES: 351; TOTAL FAT: 15G; SATURATED FAT: 3G; TRANS FAT: 0G; CHOLESTEROL: 65MG; SODIUM: 48MG; TOTAL CARBOHYDRATE: 27G; FIBER: 6G; SUGAR: 6G; PROTEIN: 29G

Sheet pan dinners make eating healthy more convenient with simple meal prep, easy cleanup, and many ways to customize your dish. This particular recipe combines green beans with baby red potatoes, which are an excellent source of the mineral potassium, which promotes healthy blood pressure, but you could use broccoli, asparagus, or sweet potatoes. An entire meal cooked on one pan, this recipe will soon become a weekly favorite when you want to keep it simple, but delicious and nutritious.

3 tablespoons olive oil, divided

4 garlic cloves, minced

2 tablespoons chopped fresh
    rosemary leaves

Salt

Freshly ground black pepper

3 cups baby red potatoes, quartered

Olive oil mister, or nonstick cooking
    spray, for preparing the pan

4 (4-ounce) boneless, skinless
    chicken breasts

1 pound fresh green beans

1 Preheat the oven to 400°F.

2 In a small bowl, whisk 2 tablespoons of olive oil, the garlic, and rosemary and season with salt and pepper.

3 In a medium bowl, toss together the potatoes and the remaining tablespoon of olive oil. Season with salt and pepper, if desired.

4 Lightly mist a large baking dish with your olive oil mister. Arrange the chicken breasts, potatoes, and green beans on the sheet. Drizzle the herbed olive oil mixture over the top. Use a pastry brush or your hands to make sure everything is evenly coated. Roast for 25 to 30 minutes, or until an instant-read thermometer in the chicken registers 165°F. The potatoes should be fork-tender, and the green beans crisp. Serve and enjoy.

Ingredient tip When watching your salt intake, you can unknowingly add more than you need when you cook. Keep in mind that 1 teaspoon of salt has almost 2,400 mg of sodium, your entire daily allowance (and far more than the low-salt goal of 1,500 per day). Be sparing and keep to a pinch, about ⅛ teaspoon, which has about 155 mg sodium.

	5 MAIN INGREDIENTS	DAIRY FREE	LOW SODIUM	NUT FREE	

Slow Cooker Hawaiian Chicken

Serves 4 | Prep time: 5 minutes | Cook time: 6 hours on low heat or 4 hours on high heat

➤ **PER SERVING** CALORIES: 244; TOTAL FAT: 4G; SATURATED FAT: 2G; TRANS FAT: 0G; CHOLESTEROL: 65MG; SODIUM: 46MG; TOTAL CARBOHYDRATE: 25G; FIBER: 1G; SUGAR: 22G; PROTEIN: 26G

This refreshing, delicious, and tropical-flavored low-cholesterol recipe is a great way to stay on track with a healthy eating plan. With fewer than 5 minutes of prep time, you can ensure that at the end of a long and busy day you will have a nutritious meal waiting for you. Pineapple is very high in the antioxidant vitamin C and has numerous anti-inflammatory phytonutrients. The sweet taste of the pineapple, slow cooked with lean chicken, creates a high-fiber dinner with an island flare.

1 pound frozen chicken breasts

1 (20-ounce) can no-sugar-added pineapple, packed in water or juice, crushed or chopped

¼ cup balsamic vinegar

2 tablespoons pure maple syrup

1 teaspoon red pepper flakes

Pinch salt

1 In a slow cooker, combine the chicken, pineapple, vinegar, maple syrup, red pepper flakes, and salt. Cover the cooker and cook for 6 hours on low heat or for 4 hours on high heat, stirring occasionally, if possible. When finished, the chicken should reach an internal temperature of 165°F and should be tender enough to tear apart easily with a fork.

2 Serve over brown rice or in lettuce wraps with a side of steamed veggies.

Ingredient tip You can use fresh pineapple in place of canned in this recipe. Look for pre-cut pineapple in the produce section of your local grocer.

	5 MAIN INGREDIENTS	BUDGET SAVER	DAIRY FREE	LOW SODIUM	NUT FREE	ONE POT	

Artichoke and Sun-Dried Tomato Chicken

Serves 4 | Prep time: 10 minutes | Cook time: 25 minutes

➤ **PER SERVING** CALORIES: 211; TOTAL FAT: 7G; SATURATED FAT: 2G; TRANS FAT: 0G; CHOLESTEROL: 65MG; SODIUM: 230MG; TOTAL CARBOHYDRATE: 10G; FIBER: 2G; SUGAR: 5G; PROTEIN: 27G

This one-pan recipe browns chicken breasts and cooks them with tasty artichoke hearts, diced tomatoes, and sun-dried tomatoes. Artichoke hearts are a delicious fit for a healthy lifestyle due to their fiber, vitamin, and mineral content. Garlic cloves add more cholesterol-lowering phytonutrients to this dish, which cooks up quickly for a speedy weeknight dinner.

4 (4-ounce) boneless, skinless chicken breasts, cut into bite-size cubes

Salt

Freshly ground black pepper

2 teaspoons olive oil

4 garlic cloves, minced

1 (14.5-ounce) can no-salt-added diced tomatoes with green peppers and onions

1 (14-ounce) can marinated artichoke hearts

⅓ cup dry-packed sun-dried tomatoes, chopped

1 Season both sides of the chicken with a scant pinch of salt and pepper. In a large skillet over medium-high heat, heat the olive oil.

2 Add the garlic. Sauté 1 to 2 minutes until softened.

3 Place the chicken in skillet. Cook for about 5 minutes per side to brown each side. Remove the chicken from pan and set aside.

4 Return the skillet to the heat. Pour the diced tomatoes into the pan. Cook for 5 minutes, stirring constantly, incorporating any browned bits from the bottom of pan.

5 Stir in the artichokes and sun-dried tomatoes, and return the chicken to the skillet. Cover the skillet and reduce the heat to medium. Simmer for 5 to 10 minutes, or until the chicken is cooked through and reaches an internal temperature of 165°F.

6 Serve over your favorite whole grain or with a side of veggies.

Substitution tip Use water-packed artichoke hearts to reduce the calories and fat content of this recipe, while keeping it flavorful with a pinch of your favorite herbs, or sauté shallots or onions with the garlic.

5 MAIN INGREDIENTS	DAIRY FREE	LOW SODIUM	NUT FREE	ONE POT

Honey Mustard Chicken

Serves 4 | Prep time: 5 minutes | Cook time: 15 minutes

➤ **PER SERVING**   CALORIES: 352; TOTAL FAT: 11G; SATURATED FAT: 3G; TRANS FAT: 0G; CHOLESTEROL: 65MG; SODIUM: 425MG; TOTAL CARBOHYDRATE: 39G; FIBER: 3G; SUGAR: 36G; PROTEIN: 28G

If you love mustard, this dinner is for you. This nutritious dish is incredibly easy to make, is ready in 20 minutes, and the honey mustard coats the chicken beautifully while clinging to the nooks and crannies of the broccoli. Because the broccoli is coated in the honey mustard it stays crisp-tender, which helps it retain more of its valuable nutrients. With lean protein and one to two servings of vegetables in each portion—nothing could be simpler.

½ cup honey, plus more as needed

¼ cup low-sodium yellow mustard, plus more as needed

¼ cup low-sodium Dijon mustard, plus more as needed

2 tablespoons olive oil

1 pound boneless, skinless chicken breast

4 cups broccoli florets

Ingredient tip Condiments such as mustard can be very high in sodium. Choose a low-salt or no-salt variety. One brand to look for is Westbrae Natural No Salt Organic Mustard. You can also make your own Dijon-style mustard: Stir together ¼ cup ground mustard with ¼ cup water and 2 tablespoons white wine vinegar. Let the mixture sit for 10 to 15 minutes before using. Refrigerate any leftovers.

1 In a medium bowl, whisk the honey with the yellow and Dijon mustards to combine. Taste and check for flavor balance, adding more honey or mustard to taste if necessary. Set aside.

2 In a large skillet over medium-high heat, heat the olive oil.

3 Add the chicken and cook for about 3 to 5 minutes per side. Cooking time will vary depending on the thickness of your chicken. The chicken should be 90 percent cooked.

4 Drizzle the honey mustard over the chicken and flip each piece a few times to coat evenly.

5 Add the broccoli and stir to combine, making sure the broccoli is coated with the honey mustard.

6 Reduce the heat to medium-low, cover the skillet, and cook for 3 to 5 minutes, steaming the broccoli until crisp-tender and cooking the chicken to an internal temperature of 165°F. Serve immediately.

5 MAIN INGREDIENTS	30 MINUTES OR FEWER	BUDGET SAVER	DAIRY FREE	LOW SODIUM	NUT FREE	

Oatmeal-Crusted Chicken Tenders

Serves 4 | Prep time: 10 minutes | Cook time: 15 minutes

➤ **PER SERVING** CALORIES: 258; TOTAL FAT: 8G; SATURATED FAT: 3G; TRANS FAT: 0G; CHOLESTEROL: 72MG; SODIUM: 210MG; TOTAL CARBOHYDRATE: 14G; FIBER: 2G; SUGAR: 1G; PROTEIN: 31G

These oatmeal-crusted chicken tenders are certain to be a hit with adults trying to reduce their cholesterol levels and children alike. Coating the chicken with whole oats adds valuable soluble fiber, while the addition of Parmesan cheese adds heart-healthy calcium. Serve these delicious tenders with your favorite veggies and dipping sauce.

1 cup old-fashioned rolled oats
½ cup freshly grated Parmesan cheese
1 teaspoon chopped fresh thyme leaves
Pinch paprika
1 pound chicken breast tenders
Salt
Freshly ground black pepper
Nonstick cooking spray

1 Preheat the oven to 450°F.

2 In a food processor, process the oats for 20 seconds until coarsely ground.

3 Add the Parmesan cheese, thyme, paprika, a pinch of salt, and pepper. Pulse to combine and transfer to a shallow bowl.

4 Place each chicken breast tender between two sheets of heavy-duty plastic wrap. Using a meat mallet or small heavy skillet, pound the chicken to a ¼-inch thickness.

5 Coat a baking sheet with cooking spray.

6 Coat both sides of the tenders with cooking spray. Dredge the tenders in the oat mixture and place them on the prepared sheet. Bake for 15 minutes, or until browned.

	5 MAIN INGREDIENTS	30 MINUTES OR FEWER	BUDGET SAVER	LOW SODIUM	NUT FREE	

Garlic-Ginger Chicken and Vegetable Stir-Fry

Serves 4 | Prep time: 5 minutes | Cook time: 20 minutes

➤ **PER SERVING** CALORIES: 216; TOTAL FAT: 7G; SATURATED FAT: 2G; TRANS FAT: 0G; CHOLESTEROL: 65MG; SODIUM: 58MG; TOTAL CARBOHYDRATE: 8G; FIBER: 2G; SUGAR: 7G; PROTEIN: 26G

After making this recipe you will put that Chinese takeout menu in the back of the drawer. This recipe is low in fat and high in fiber and essential vitamins and minerals. It's also low in sodium because spices and garlic provide flavor, rather than the high-sodium salt or soy sauce often used by restaurants. You can easily personalize this recipe by adding different spices and additional veggies.

1 tablespoon sesame oil

1 pound boneless, skinless chicken breasts or tenders, cut into 1-inch cubes

4 garlic cloves, minced

2 tablespoons brown sugar

2 tablespoons grated, peeled fresh ginger

1 (16-ounce) package frozen stir-fry vegetables

Low-sodium soy sauce, for serving (optional)

Chopped fresh cilantro, for serving (optional)

1 In a large saucepan or wok over medium-high heat, heat the sesame oil.

2 Add the chicken and garlic. Cook for 2 to 3 minutes, stirring constantly, until the chicken is lightly browned.

3 Stir in the brown sugar and ginger. Cook for 2 to 3 minutes more, until the ginger is browned.

4 Add the stir-fry vegetables and reduce the heat to medium. Cover the pan and cook for 10 to 15 minutes, stirring occasionally.

5 Serve over brown rice, whole-wheat noodles, or quinoa with a dash of low-sodium soy sauce and sprinkling of cilantro, if desired.

Substitution tip Sesame oil gives the stir-fry a deep, rich flavor, which is hard to replicate with a substitute. However, you could use peanut oil or olive oil and a couple tablespoons of chopped peanuts as a garnish.

5 MAIN INGREDIENTS	30 MINUTES OR FEWER	BUDGET SAVER	DAIRY FREE	LOW SODIUM	NUT FREE	ONE POT

Slow Cooker Turkey and Chickpea Chili

Serves 6 | Prep time: 5 minutes | Cook time: 4 to 6 hours on low heat or 2 hours on high heat

➤ PER SERVING   CALORIES: 290; TOTAL FAT: 2G; SATURATED FAT: 0G; TRANS FAT: 0G; CHOLESTEROL: 93MG; SODIUM: 294MG; TOTAL CARBOHYDRATE: 24G; FIBER: 7G; SUGAR: 8G; PROTEIN: 44G

Slow cooker chili dishes are perfect in fall and winter when you're craving a hot, nourishing, comforting meal. This turkey chili recipe is different from most in that it uses lean turkey breast, slow cooked with soluble fiber–rich chickpeas, for a creative slow cooker recipe that is healthy and delicious. Freeze leftovers so you have a healthy meal on hand when you are pressed for time.

4 cups boneless, skinless turkey breast, cut into strips (from about 1½ pounds)

2 (14-ounce) cans no-salt-added diced tomatoes

1 (15-ounce) can chickpeas, drained and rinsed

1 (10-ounce) package frozen spinach

1 (6-ounce) can diced green chilies

1 small onion, diced

2 cups low-sodium chicken broth

2 garlic cloves, minced

1 tablespoon chili powder

1 teaspoon ground cumin

½ teaspoon freshly ground black pepper

1 In a 6-quart slow cooker, combine the turkey, tomatoes, chickpeas, spinach, green chilies, onion, chicken broth, garlic, chili powder, cumin, and pepper. Stir to combine.

2 Cover the cooker and cook for 4 to 6 hours on low heat or for 2 hours on high heat, until the turkey reaches an internal temperature of 165°F. Serve hot.

DAIRY FREE	LOW SODIUM	NUT FREE	ONE POT

Wholesome Turkey Meatloaf

Serves 4 | Prep time: 10 minutes | Cook time: 55 minutes

➤ **PER SERVING** CALORIES: 233; TOTAL FAT: 7G; SATURATED FAT: 1G; TRANS FAT: 0G; CHOLESTEROL: 102MG; SODIUM: 185MG; TOTAL CARBOHYDRATE: 13G; FIBER: 2G; SUGAR: 3G; PROTEIN: 30G

While traditional meatloaf recipes can be high in sodium, calories, and unhealthy fats, it is surprisingly easy to keep the flavor while boosting the nutritional content. This recipe uses lean ground turkey instead of beef, and swaps out bread crumbs for toasted whole-grain bread, while reducing the use of processed condiments. This is a great recipe to double, as cooked slices are perfect to freeze so you have something homemade on hand when you just don't feel like cooking.

1 tablespoon olive oil

1 cup small-dice yellow onion

4 garlic cloves, minced

1 pound lean or extra-lean ground turkey

2 slices whole-grain bread, broken into small crumbs

1 large egg, or ¼ cup liquid egg white, beaten

¼ teaspoon freshly ground black pepper

Sliced scallions, for garnish (optional)

Salsa, for garnish (optional)

Ketchup, for garnish (optional)

1 Preheat the oven to 350°F.

2 In a medium pan over medium-high heat, heat the olive oil.

3 Add the onion and garlic. Cook for about 5 minutes, stirring occasionally, until softened. Transfer to a large bowl. Let cool for 5 minutes.

4 Mix the turkey, bread, egg, and pepper with the onion-garlic mixture. Shape into a loaf and place in a glass baking dish. Bake for 50 to 55 minutes, or until an instant-read thermometer registers 165°F.

5 Remove from the oven and top as desired. Serve hot.

Substitution tip You can put anything you want into a meatloaf. For more fiber and cholesterol-lowering nutrients, add chopped spinach, mushrooms, tomatoes, or your favorite veggies to the recipe. Depending on the type of veggie used, you may want to sauté them lightly along with the onion and garlic.

	5 MAIN INGREDIENTS	DAIRY FREE	LOW SODIUM	NUT FREE	

Glazed Turkey Cutlets and Bell Peppers

Serves 4 | Prep time: 5 minutes | Cook time: 15 minutes

➤ **PER SERVING** CALORIES: 171; TOTAL FAT: 3G; SATURATED FAT: 0G; TRANS FAT: 0G; CHOLESTEROL: 70MG; SODIUM: 59MG; TOTAL CARBOHYDRATE: 8G; FIBER: 1G; SUGAR: 4G; PROTEIN: 29G

Turkey cutlets are an economical, flavorful, and lean meat, cut from the turkey breast. Because they are typically thin, they take well to marinades and cook quickly, without a chance of drying out. Used in this colorful recipe with fiber- and vitamin C–rich peppers, the turkey cutlets are topped with a balsamic glaze.

3 tablespoons balsamic vinegar

2 teaspoons honey

¼ cup water

1 pound ¼-inch-thick turkey breast cutlets

Freshly ground black pepper

Salt

2 teaspoons olive oil

2 garlic cloves, minced

2 red bell peppers, seeded and cut into strips

1 In a small bowl, whisk the vinegar, honey, and water. Set aside.

2 Season both sides of the turkey cutlets with pepper and a scant pinch of salt.

3 In a large nonstick skillet over medium-high heat, heat the olive oil until hot.

4 Add the garlic. Sauté for 30 seconds until fragrant.

5 Add the turkey. Cook for 2 minutes per side, or until done, reaching an internal temperature of 165°F. Remove the cutlets from the skillet and keep warm.

6 Return the skillet to the heat, reduce the heat to medium, and add the red bell peppers. Sauté for 2 minutes.

7 Stir in the balsamic mixture and cook for 3 minutes, stirring constantly, until reduced by about half.

8 Spoon the sauce and red bell peppers over the cutlets. Serve with brown rice or your favorite whole grain.

Substitution tip If you have low-sodium chicken broth on hand, replace the water with ¼ cup broth to boost the flavor even further.

5 MAIN INGREDIENTS	30 MINUTES OR FEWER	DAIRY FREE	LOW SODIUM	NUT FREE

Rosemary Turkey Cutlets with Shallots and Zucchini

Serves 4 | Prep time: 5 minutes | Cook time: 15 minutes

➤ PER SERVING   CALORIES: 209; TOTAL FAT: 8G; SATURATED FAT: 1G; TRANS FAT: 0G; CHOLESTEROL: 70MG; SODIUM: 73MG; TOTAL CARBOHYDRATE: 6G; FIBER: 2G; SUGAR: 2G; PROTEIN: 29G

Rosemary is a fragrant evergreen herb that not only tastes delicious, but is also a good source of vitamins and minerals, and powerful inflammation-reducing antioxidants. Intensely flavored, rosemary pairs well with the hearty taste of turkey. Shallots add their unique flavor in addition to the phytonutrient, allicin, which may reduce cholesterol levels. Serve this boldly flavored dish with a side of roasted sweet potatoes.

2 tablespoons olive oil, divided

4 (4-ounce) boneless, skinless turkey breast cutlets

Salt

Freshly ground black pepper

4 shallots, quartered lengthwise

2 medium zucchini, sliced (about 2 cups)

8 (1-inch) rosemary sprigs

¾ cup low-sodium chicken broth

1 In a large skillet over medium-high heat, heat 1 tablespoon of olive oil.

2 Season the turkey cutlets with salt and pepper. Place them in the skillet and cook for 1 to 2 minutes per side until browned. Transfer to a plate.

3 Return the skillet to the heat. Add the remaining tablespoon of olive oil and the shallots. Cook for about 4 minutes, stirring occasionally, until the shallots begin to soften.

4 Add the zucchini and cook for 2 minutes until softened.

5 Stir in the rosemary and chicken broth. Cook for about 2 minutes until reduced by half.

6 Return the turkey to the skillet and cook for about 1 minute until warmed through. Remove from the heat and serve.

	5 MAIN INGREDIENTS	30 MINUTES OR FEWER	DAIRY FREE	LOW SODIUM	NUT FREE	ONE POT	

Southwestern Turkey-Quinoa Skillet

Serves 4 | Prep time: 10 minutes | Cook time: 35 minutes

➤ **PER SERVING** CALORIES: 280; TOTAL FAT: 3G; SATURATED FAT: 0G; TRANS FAT: 0G; CHOLESTEROL: 28MG; SODIUM: 100MG; TOTAL CARBOHYDRATE: 43G; FIBER: 9G; SUGAR: 7G; PROTEIN: 23G

Skillet meals are a great time-saver when you want to eat healthy but don't want to spend all night in the kitchen. Simple, yet packed with nutrition and flavor, this easy recipe uses lean ground turkey, and a colorful mix of fiber-, vitamin-, and mineral-rich beans, veggies, and quinoa. Serve this Southwestern skillet in a bowl topped with avocado, rolled up in a corn tortilla with salsa, or as a salad topping.

Nonstick cooking spray

8 ounces 99% lean ground turkey

2 garlic cloves, minced

2 teaspoons chili powder

1 teaspoon ground cumin

1 (15-ounce) can black beans, drained and rinsed

1 (14.5-ounce) can no-salt-added, fire-roasted diced tomatoes

½ cup frozen corn

½ cup quinoa, rinsed

½ cup water

1 Generously spray a large skillet with cooking spray and place it over medium-high heat. When the skillet is hot, add the ground turkey and garlic. Cook for about 5 minutes until the meat is almost cooked through, breaking it up with a spoon as it cooks.

2 Stir in the chili powder, cumin, black beans, tomatoes, corn, and quinoa, stirring until everything is combined. When the mixture starts to bubble, add the water, cover the skillet, and reduce the heat to medium-low. Simmer for 20 to 25 minutes until most of the liquid is absorbed and the quinoa is cooked. Serve hot.

DAIRY FREE	LOW SODIUM	NUT FREE	ONE POT

Turkey Cutlets with Parmesan Crust

Serves 4 | Prep time: 10 minutes | Cook time: 15 minutes

➤ **PER SERVING**   CALORIES: 193; TOTAL FAT: 5G; SATURATED FAT: 1G; TRANS FAT: 0G; CHOLESTEROL: 72MG; SODIUM: 137MG; TOTAL CARBOHYDRATE: 5G; FIBER: 1G; SUGAR: 0G; PROTEIN: 32G

If chicken is your fallback protein, you may be interested to learn that turkey breast is slightly lower in calories, total fat, and cholesterol. It's a great choice for a healthy dinner, and simple and delicious to prepare. These garlic-Parmesan turkey breast cutlets are a tasty main dish packed with flavor and quick to fix. Serve with your favorite sides.

4 (4-ounce) turkey breast cutlets

Salt

Freshly ground black pepper

⅓ cup whole-wheat panko
   bread crumbs

2 tablespoons grated Parmesan cheese

2 teaspoons dried parsley

2 large egg whites, beaten

1 tablespoon olive oil

Lemon wedges, for serving (optional)

Chopped fresh parsley leaves,
   for serving (optional)

1 Season the cutlets with salt and pepper.

2 In a medium bowl, stir together the bread crumbs, Parmesan cheese, and dried parsley.

3 In another bowl beat the egg whites.

4 Heat a large nonstick skillet over medium heat.

5 Dip the turkey cutlets in the egg whites and into the bread crumb mixture, shaking off any excess.

6 Add the olive oil to the skillet, followed by the breaded cutlets. Cook for about 6 minutes per side, until golden brown and cooked to an internal temperature of 165°F. Serve with lemon wedges and fresh parsley (if using).

	5 MAIN INGREDIENTS	30 MINUTES OR FEWER	BUDGET SAVER	LOW SODIUM	NUT FREE	

Sautéed Turkey Cutlets with Avocado Sauce

Serves 4 | Prep time: 5 minutes | Cook time: 10 minutes

➤ **PER SERVING** CALORIES: 435; TOTAL FAT: 25G; SATURATED FAT: 3G; TRANS FAT: 0G; CHOLESTEROL: 70MG; SODIUM: 62MG; TOTAL CARBOHYDRATE: 25G; FIBER: 9G; SUGAR: 0G; PROTEIN: 33G

Sometimes all you need to add variety to your healthy eating plan is a creative and delicious nutrient-dense sauce to smother your lean protein. This recipe uses delectable avocado to make a fiber-full and heart-healthy, monounsaturated fat–rich sauce for lightly sautéed turkey breasts. Uncomplicated and full of cholesterol-lowering nutrients, serve this main dish with your favorite sides.

FOR THE AVOCADO SAUCE

2 medium ripe avocados
(about 1 pound),
halved and pitted
2 garlic cloves
2 tablespoons water, plus more
as needed
2 tablespoons freshly squeezed lime
juice (about 1 lime)
1 tablespoon olive oil

FOR THE TURKEY

¾ cup oat flour
Salt
Freshly ground black pepper
4 (4-ounce) boneless, skinless turkey
breast cutlets
1 tablespoon olive oil
Fresh basil leaves, for garnish (optional)

TO MAKE THE AVOCADO SAUCE

Scoop the avocado flesh into a blender and add the garlic, water, lime juice, and olive oil. Process until smooth. Set aside until ready to use. If the sauce is too thick, add a little more water.

TO MAKE THE TURKEY

1 In a shallow dish or resealable plastic bag, combine the flour with the salt and pepper. Mix thoroughly.

2 Add half of the cutlets, seal the bag, and shake to coat well. Remove the cutlets, shake off any excess flour, and set aside. Repeat with the remaining cutlets.

3 In a large skillet over medium heat, heat the olive oil until it shimmers.

4 Add the cutlets. Cook for 1 to 2 minutes per side until browned, or until they reach an internal temperature of 165°F.

5 Top the turkey cutlets with the avocado sauce and garnish with torn basil leaves (if using).

5 MAIN INGREDIENTS	30 MINUTES OR FEWER	BUDGET SAVER	LOW SODIUM	NUT FREE

Turkey Cutlets with Brussels Sprouts and Cranberries

Serves 4 | Prep time: 5 minutes | Cook time: 15 minutes

➤ **PER SERVING** CALORIES: 261; TOTAL FAT: 11G; SATURATED FAT: 2G; TRANS FAT: 0G; CHOLESTEROL: 70MG; SODIUM: 84MG; TOTAL CARBOHYDRATE: 11G; FIBER: 2G; SUGAR: 7G; PROTEIN: 30G

Reminiscent of Thanksgiving, this dish is a medley of holiday favorites, with lean, high-quality protein, accompanied by fiber- and antioxidant-rich Brussels sprouts and cranberries. A one-pot meal that tastes like you went to a lot of trouble, this easy recipe comes together quickly to produce a moist and flavorful balanced meal.

3 tablespoons olive oil, divided

4 (4-ounce) boneless, skinless turkey breast cutlets

Salt

Freshly ground black pepper

8 ounces Brussels sprouts, trimmed, quartered through the root end

¾ cup low-sodium chicken broth

¼ cup unsweetened dried cranberries

1 tablespoon chopped fresh sage leaves

Salt

Freshly ground black pepper

1½ teaspoons red wine vinegar (optional)

1 In a large skillet over medium-high heat, heat 2 tablespoons of olive oil.

2 Season the turkey cutlets with salt and pepper and add them to the skillet. Sauté for about 3 minutes per side, until golden brown and cooked through to an internal temperature of 165°F. Transfer to a plate and tent with aluminum foil to keep warm.

3 Return the skillet to the heat, and add the remaining tablespoon of olive oil, the Brussels sprouts, chicken broth, cranberries, and sage. Cover the skillet and cook for about 5 minutes, until the Brussels sprouts are crisp-tender, stirring occasionally. Season with salt and pepper, and stir in the vinegar (if using).

4 Spoon the Brussels sprouts mixture over the turkey cutlets and serve.

Ingredient tip The vinegar is not essential to this recipe, but it adds a slight acidity and some sweetness.

5 MAIN INGREDIENTS	30 MINUTES OR FEWER	DAIRY FREE	LOW SODIUM	NUT FREE	ONE POT

Mediterranean Turkey Kebabs

Serves 4 | Prep time: 1 hour, 10 minutes | Cook time: 20 minutes

➤ **PER SERVING** CALORIES: 240; TOTAL FAT: 8G; SATURATED FAT: 1G; TRANS FAT: 0G; CHOLESTEROL: 70MG; SODIUM: 69MG; TOTAL CARBOHYDRATE: 15G; FIBER: 2G; SUGAR: 7G; PROTEIN: 29G

Kebabs are a fun and colorful way to create a meal on a stick, and one that's adaptable to just about any protein, fruit, or vegetable. This particular recipe gets you out of your chicken or steak rut with turkey breast and Mediterranean vegetables. Feel free to use whatever veggies you have on hand and mix up the spices based on your favorites.

½ cup balsamic vinegar

2 tablespoons olive oil, plus more for the grill

1 tablespoon honey

1 pound boneless, skinless turkey breast cutlets, cut into 2-inch pieces

2 large zucchini, cut into 1-inch pieces

1 large onion, cut into 1-inch pieces

1 Soak 8 (10-inch) wooden skewers in water for 30 minutes. Alternatively, use metal skewers, no soaking required!

2 While the skewers soak, whisk the vinegar, olive oil, and honey in a small bowl. Set aside.

3 Onto each skewer, thread 2 pieces of turkey, 2 zucchini pieces, and 1 onion piece. Place the kebabs in a shallow dish and pour the marinade over. Cover with plastic wrap and refrigerate to marinate for 1 hour, turning occasionally.

4 Prepare a grill, or grill pan, for high heat.

5 Drain the marinade from the kebabs and reserve the marinade.

6 Lightly oil the grill grate. Place the skewers on the grill, close the cover, and cook for 14 to 16 minutes until the juices run clear, turning twice.

7 In a medium saucepan over high heat, bring the reserved marinade to a boil. Boil for 1 minute. Remove from the heat and drizzle the marinade over the skewers.

	5 MAIN INGREDIENTS	DAIRY FREE	LOW SODIUM	NUT FREE	

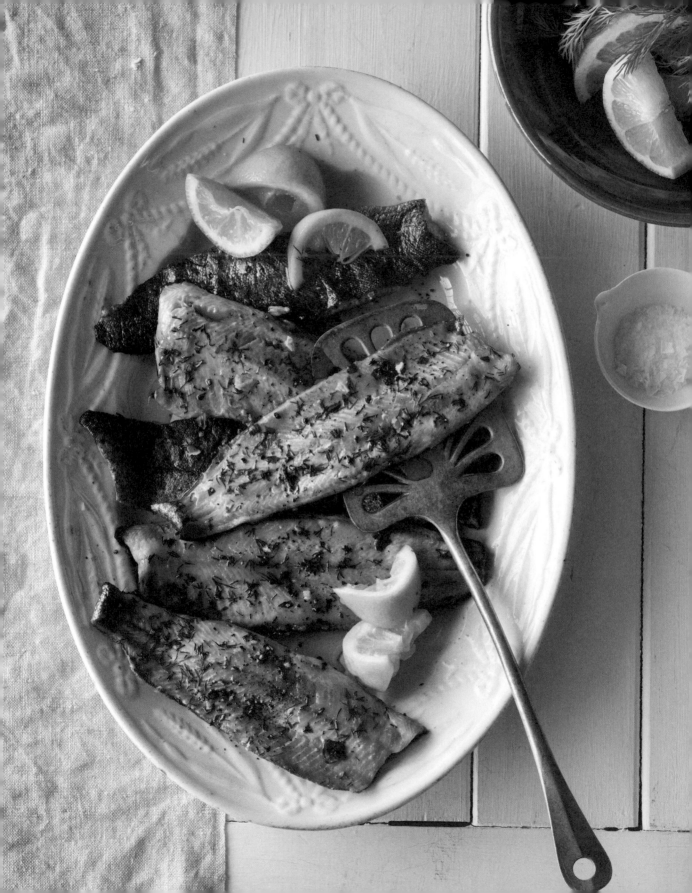

CHAPTER 7

Seafood Mains

Yogurt-Marinated Grilled Salmon

Serves 4 | Prep time: 5 minutes | Marinating time: 1 hour to overnight | Cook time: 8 minutes

➤ **PER SERVING**   CALORIES: 182; TOTAL FAT: 5G; SATURATED FAT: 1G; TRANS FAT: 0G; CHOLESTEROL: 69MG; SODIUM: 136MG; TOTAL CARBOHYDRATE: 7G; FIBER: 2G; SUGAR: 2G; PROTEIN: 28G

Salmon is an excellent source of heart-healthy omega-3 fatty acids, and is also high in vitamin D, a nutrient that is low in the diets of many Americans. The AHA recommends consuming fish twice per week to lower your risk for heart disease. This simple, tasty recipe uses a yogurt marinade, which produces a silky texture. Marinating the fish overnight allows the flavors to really penetrate the fish, but if you are pressed for time, one hour will do.

1 cup plain low-fat Greek yogurt

1 tablespoon Sriracha

4 (4-ounce) boneless, skinless
   salmon fillets

½ cup chopped fresh cilantro

1 lemon, cut into wedges

Did you know? One serving of salmon is 2 to 3 ounces. A salmon steak is usually between 4 and 6 ounces, or about two servings, but keep in mind that fish and meats shrink about 25 percent when cooked, so purchasing a 4- to 6-ounce raw steak will result in an appropriate serving size. According to the USDA, women should consume about 5 ounces of protein daily; men, 6 ounces; and children, 2 to 5 ounces depending on age.

1 In a large bowl, whisk the yogurt and Sriracha.

2 Add the salmon and turn to coat. Cover the bowl with plastic wrap and refrigerate for 1 to 8 hours, or overnight.

3 Prepare a grill for medium-high heat.

4 Remove the salmon from the marinade and discard the excess marinade. Arrange the salmon on the grill grates or in a fish basket. Close the cover and cook for 4 minutes. Gently turn the salmon and continue cooking or 4 more minutes, until the salmon is cooked through and flakes easily with a fork. Alternatively, bake the salmon on a parchment paper–lined baking sheet at 400°F for 12 to 15 minutes, until cooked through to an internal temperature of 145°F and the salmon flakes easily with a fork. Transfer the salmon to plates or a platter. Sprinkle with cilantro and serve with lemon wedges.

5 MAIN INGREDIENTS	LOW SODIUM	NUT FREE

Baked Flounder Packets with Summer Squash

Serves 4 | Prep time: 15 minutes | Cook time: 15 minutes

➤ **PER SERVING** CALORIES: 182; TOTAL FAT: 8G; SATURATED FAT: 1G; TRANS FAT: 0G; CHOLESTEROL: 48MG; SODIUM: 89MG; TOTAL CARBOHYDRATE: 7G; FIBER: 3G; SUGAR: 2G; PROTEIN: 22G

This no-fuss dish of flounder in aluminum foil packets with summer squash is one of the easiest recipes to prepare, clean up, and scale. The recipe works whether you are cooking for two, four, or a crowd. The fish and vegetables steam inside individual foil packets, making this a quick-cooking main course that's easy to customize with your favorite fish, veggies, and herbs. Serve with brown rice or roasted sweet potatoes.

4 (4-ounce) flounder fillets, or other white-fleshed fish
Freshly ground black pepper
Salt
2 zucchini, thinly sliced
1 yellow squash, thinly sliced
1 medium red onion, sliced
2 tablespoons olive oil
8 thyme sprigs
Lemon wedges, for serving (optional)

Did you know? Parchment or foil for cooking fish packets? Either works fine, but if you have parchment, the packet will brown attractively and also puff up a bit in the oven. Using parchment for delicate, thin, white-fleshed fish is particularly delicious.

1 Preheat the oven to 450°F.

2 Season the fish with pepper and a pinch of salt.

3 Arrange 4 large sheets of foil on a work surface. Place one fillet on each piece of foil.

4 Arrange some of the zucchini, squash, and red onion around each fillet, and drizzle 1½ teaspoons of olive oil onto each piece of fish and the vegetables. Place two thyme sprigs on each fillet.

5 Wrap the foil around the fish and vegetables, leaving some air space within each packet, and seal them very well. Set the packets on a rimmed baking sheet and bake for 15 minutes. Carefully open one packet, being careful of the hot steam escaping, and confirm that the fish is cooked through to an internal temperature of 145°F and flakes easily with a fork. If not, reseal the packet and return it to the oven to continue cooking until cooked through.

6 Serve immediately, opening the packets at the table, and serve with lemon wedges (if using).

5 MAIN INGREDIENTS	30 MINUTES OR FEWER	DAIRY FREE	LOW SODIUM	NUT FREE	ONE POT

Steamed Rosemary Trout in Parchment with Spinach

Serves 4 | Prep time: 10 minutes | Cook time: 15 minutes

> ➤ **PER SERVING** CALORIES: 257; TOTAL FAT: 11G; SATURATED FAT: 3G; TRANS FAT: 0G; CHOLESTEROL: 78MG; SODIUM: 95MG; TOTAL CARBOHYDRATE: 9G; FIBER: 4G; SUGAR: 1G; PROTEIN: 32G

This simple, yet delicious trout en papillote (cooked and served in a paper wrapper) is made with a mix of fiber- and nutrient-rich spinach and mushrooms, with the bold flavor of rosemary. Omega-3 fatty acid content varies depending on the type of trout, with lake trout topping the list with even higher amounts than salmon. All trout has significant amounts of omega-3 fats, however; so choose the type that is most readily available.

2 cups (about 5 ounces) fresh baby spinach

4 small (4-ounce) rainbow trout, cleaned and boned (use fillets if whole trout are not available)

Salt

Freshly ground black pepper

4 portobello mushroom caps, thinly sliced

4 shallots, chopped

1 tablespoon olive oil

4 rosemary sprigs

1 Preheat the oven to 450°F.

2 Cut 4 sheets of parchment paper or aluminum foil into squares that are 3 inches longer than your fish.

3 Pile one-fourth of the spinach leaves in the middle of each piece. Lay one fish fillet on each bed of spinach. Season with salt and pepper.

4 Layer each fish with mushroom slices.

	5 MAIN INGREDIENTS	30 MINUTES OR FEWER	DAIRY FREE	LOW SODIUM	NUT FREE	

5 In a small bowl, stir together the shallots and olive oil. Spoon the shallots over the middle of each piece of fish, and top each with 1 rosemary sprig. Make sure the trout are in the middle of each square, fold the packet up around the fish, and crimp together tightly to seal. Place the packets on a baking sheet and bake for 10 to 15 minutes, checking one packet after 10 minutes. The flesh should be opaque and pull apart easily when testing with a fork.

6 Place each packet on a plate and carefully open, being aware of the hot steam escaping. Gently remove the fish from the packet and pour the juices over. Serve immediately with steamed brown rice or your favorite whole grain.

Substitution tip While working to lower your cholesterol level through dietary changes, make it a habit always to include a couple garlic cloves and some shallots and/or onions with every meal. This habit ensures that each day you get the phytonutrient allicin, a powerful cholesterol-lowering nutrient.

Trout with Herbs and Lemon

Serves 6 | Prep time: 5 minutes | Cook time: 15 minutes

➤ **PER SERVING** CALORIES: 183; TOTAL FAT: 12G; SATURATED FAT: 2G; TRANS FAT: 0G; CHOLESTEROL: 45MG; SODIUM: 261MG; TOTAL CARBOHYDRATE: 7G; FIBER: 2G; SUGAR: 0G; PROTEIN: 16G

If you find salmon a bit too rich for your taste, you might consider trout. Equally high in heart-healthy omega-3 fatty acids, trout has a mild, sweet fish taste and less of an "oily" taste than salmon. Trout can be prepared very simply, as in this quick recipe, with lemon and dill as the major companions. Serve with your favorite vegetables and grain.

Juice of 2 lemons

1 small bunch fresh dill, finely snipped

2 tablespoons plus 2 teaspoons
   olive oil, divided

6 (3-ounce) trout fillets

Salt

Freshly ground black pepper

2 lemons, sliced

1 Preheat the oven to 400°F.

2 In a small bowl, stir together the lemon juice, dill, and 2 tablespoons olive oil.

3 Using the remaining 2 teaspoons of olive oil, lightly grease a shallow glass casserole dish and place the trout skin-side down in the dish.

4 Pour the lemon-dill mixture over the fish to coat. Season with salt and pepper and top with the lemon slices. Roast the fish for about 12 minutes, until the flesh turns a soft coral shade and flakes easily with a fork. Serve with your favorite sides.

5 MAIN INGREDIENTS	30 MINUTES OR FEWER	DAIRY FREE	LOW SODIUM	NUT FREE

Arctic Char with Cherry Tomatoes

Serves 4 | Prep time: 5 minutes | Cook time: 15 minutes

➤ **PER SERVING** CALORIES: 234; TOTAL FAT: 11G; SATURATED FAT: 2G; TRANS FAT: 0G; CHOLESTEROL: 45MG; SODIUM: 84MG; TOTAL CARBOHYDRATE: 8G; FIBER: 1G; SUGAR: 2G; PROTEIN: 20G

Arctic char is a flavorful, pink-fleshed fish that is related to trout and salmon, and resembles salmon, but with a more colorful body. Arctic char tastes like a cross between trout and salmon, and it provides high amounts of the carotenoid antioxidant phytonutrients and omega-3 fatty acids. If your local grocer doesn't stock char, substitute salmon. This recipe bakes the char while fresh cherry tomatoes are lightly sautéed with fresh basil. Serve with your favorite whole grain or steamed potatoes.

4 (4- to 6-ounce) arctic char fillets

Salt

Freshly ground black pepper

4 teaspoons plus 1 tablespoon olive oil, divided

4 shallots, minced

1 red onion, sliced

2 cups cherry tomatoes

¼ cup thinly sliced fresh basil leaves

1 Preheat the oven to 450°F.

2 Line a baking sheet with parchment paper.

3 Season the fillets with salt and pepper, and rub each with 1 teaspoon of olive oil. Place on the prepared sheet and bake for 12 to 15 minutes, or until your desired doneness.

4 Meanwhile, heat a large nonstick skillet over medium heat. Add the remaining tablespoon of olive oil to pan and swirl to coat.

5 Add the shallots and red onion. Cook for 2 minutes, or until lightly browned, stirring occasionally. Increase the heat to medium-high.

6 Add tomatoes to the skillet and sauté for 2 minutes, or until the skins blister, stirring frequently. Remove the pan from the heat. Season the tomato mixture with salt and pepper and fresh basil. Toss to combine. Serve the tomatoes over the fish.

5 MAIN INGREDIENTS	30 MINUTES OR FEWER	DAIRY FREE	LOW SODIUM	NUT FREE

Shrimp Scampi with Spinach and Lemon

Serves 2 | Prep time: 5 minutes | Cook time: 15 minutes

➤ **PER SERVING** CALORIES: 540; TOTAL FAT: 18G; SATURATED FAT: 2G; TRANS FAT: 0G; CHOLESTEROL: 212MG; SODIUM: 377MG; TOTAL CARBOHYDRATE: 54G; FIBER: 10G; SUGAR: 5G; PROTEIN: 37G

Many people seeking to lower their cholesterol levels avoid shrimp due to its relatively high content of dietary cholesterol. However, dietary cholesterol does not raise your body's cholesterol; instead, it is the saturated fats and trans fats in the diet that do. Shrimp are very low in calories and saturated and trans fats, so enjoy them freely in your cholesterol-lowering plan. This healthy scampi uses whole-wheat angel hair pasta to boost the overall fiber content.

8 ounces whole-wheat angel hair pasta

2 tablespoons olive oil

8 ounces large shrimp, peeled and deveined

4 shallots, minced

4 cups fresh baby spinach

Red pepper flakes, for seasoning (optional)

¼ cup dry white wine

Salt

Freshly ground black pepper

Juice of 1 lemon

Freshly grated Parmesan cheese, for garnish (optional)

Ingredient tip If you like a richer-tasting dish, add 1 tablespoon margarine to the skillet before adding the shrimp back to the pan. Consider purchasing a soft margarine with added plant stanols, which are plant phytonutrients shown to lower cholesterol levels. One brand to look for is Benecol.

1 Cook the pasta according to the package directions. Drain, reserving the cooking water, and set aside.

2 In a large heavy skillet over medium-high heat, heat the olive oil until it shimmers.

3 Add the shrimp. Sauté for about 1 minute per side until just barely cooked through. Transfer the shrimp to a plate.

4 Return the skillet to the heat and add the shallots, spinach, and red pepper flakes (if using). Sauté for about 1 minute, until the spinach begins to wilt.

5 Add the wine, and salt and pepper. Reduce the heat to medium and cook for 1 to 2 minutes.

6 Return the shrimp to the skillet and remove it from the heat.

7 Toss the cooked pasta with the shrimp and spinach in the skillet, adding the reserved water if needed to moisten.

8 Squeeze the lemon juice over the skillet and sprinkle with Parmesan cheese (if using).

30 MINUTES OR FEWER	LOW SODIUM	NUT FREE

Walnut-Crusted Halibut

Serves 4 | Prep time: 10 minutes | Cook time: 10 minutes

➤ **PER SERVING** CALORIES: 359; TOTAL FAT: 28G; SATURATED FAT: 3G; TRANS FAT: 0G; CHOLESTEROL: 40MG; SODIUM: 76MG; TOTAL CARBOHYDRATE: 5G; FIBER: 2G; SUGAR: 1G; PROTEIN: 28G

One way to incorporate more nuts into your diet is to use them as a coating for baked fish. Nuts, especially walnuts and almonds, are rich in heart-healthy fats, and important vitamins and minerals. Using nuts in place of regular bread crumbs gives you more nutrition for about the same amount of calories. You can use any type of fish or nut in this recipe. For a complete meal, add some vegetables and potatoes to the pan to roast along with the fish.

Nonstick cooking spray

1½ cups finely chopped walnuts

1 tablespoon lemon zest

1 teaspoon dried dill

Salt

Freshly ground black pepper

4 (4- to 6-ounce) halibut fillets, skin removed

2 tablespoons olive oil, divided

Lemon wedges, for serving

1 Preheat the oven to 450°F.

2 Spray a rimmed baking sheet with cooking spray.

3 In a small bowl, mix together the walnuts, lemon zest, and dill. Season with salt and pepper.

4 Brush each fillet with 1½ teaspoons of olive oil and sprinkle with salt and pepper. Place the fish on the prepared sheet. Sprinkle the walnut mixture atop the fish, dividing equally and pressing to adhere. Roast the fish for about 8 minutes, until just opaque in the center. If a crispier topping is desired, preheat the broiler and broil the fish for about 1 minute, watching carefully to prevent burning. Transfer the fish to plates and serve with the lemon wedges.

Ingredient tip To chop walnuts finely, place them in a clean coffee grinder or mini food prep food processor. Alternatively, use a chef's knife with a large tapered blade. Grasp the handle and place your other hand over the tip. Carefully rock the blade across the nuts until the pieces are your desired size.

5 MAIN INGREDIENTS	30 MINUTES OR FEWER	DAIRY FREE	LOW SODIUM

Ginger-Lemon Cod with Roasted Broccoli and Rice

Serves 4 | Prep time: 10 minutes | Cook time: 25 minutes

➤ **PER SERVING** CALORIES: 342; TOTAL FAT: 12G; SATURATED FAT: 2G; TRANS FAT: 0G; CHOLESTEROL: 40MG; SODIUM: 121MG; TOTAL CARBOHYDRATE: 30G; FIBER: 7G; SUGAR: 3G; PROTEIN: 26G

This simple, tangy fish dish is seasoned with ginger and lemon, and cooked quickly by pan searing. Ginger contains a powerful substance called gingerol that can reduce inflammation in the body, and it gives the dish a spicy bite while imparting its beneficial nutrients. For a complete meal, nutrient-rich broccoli is roasted to accompany the fish.

1 pound broccoli, cut into florets

3 tablespoons olive oil, divided

Salt

Freshly ground black pepper

1 cup instant brown rice

1 tablespoon grated peeled fresh ginger

2 garlic cloves, grated

2 lemons, sliced

4 (4- to 6-ounce) cod fillets

½ cup dry white wine

¼ cup fresh chives, chopped, plus more for garnishing (optional)

1 Preheat the oven to 450°F.

2 Line a sheet pan with parchment paper and put the broccoli florets on the pan. Drizzle with 1 tablespoon of olive oil and season with salt and pepper. Bake for about 20 minutes, until golden brown.

3 Meanwhile, cook the brown rice according to the package directions.

4 In a small bowl, stir together 1 tablespoon of olive oil, the ginger, garlic, and lemon slices. Season with salt and pepper and set aside.

5 In a large skillet over medium-high heat, heat the remaining tablespoon of olive oil until it shimmers.

6 Add the fish to the skillet. Sear for 5 minutes. Move the fish to the side of the skillet, stacking them as needed and leaving room in the center of the pan.

	DAIRY FREE	LOW SODIUM	NUT FREE	

7 Add the ginger-lemon mixture and sauté for about 3 minutes until the lemon slices are golden brown.

8 Add the white wine and chives. Cook for about 3 minutes, stirring, until a sauce begins to form. Scoop some of the sauce over the fish.

9 Stir the rice into the pan and cook until the sauce is fully absorbed.

10 Transfer the fish to serving plates, portion the sauced rice next to the fish, and top with roasted broccoli. Garnish with additional chives, if desired.

Did you know? The nutritional difference between a serving of long-grain brown rice, which requires 35 to 45 minutes to cook, and instant brown rice, which cooks in 5 minutes, is insignificant. Instant rice has simply been cooked and dehydrated so it cooks quicker than long-grain rice.

Salmon Skewers with Yogurt Sauce

Serves 4 | Prep time: 25 minutes | Cook time: 10 minutes

➤ **PER SERVING** CALORIES: 643; TOTAL FAT: 39G; SATURATED FAT: 6G; TRANS FAT: 0G; CHOLESTEROL: 120MG; SODIUM: 700MG; TOTAL CARBOHYDRATE: 30G; FIBER: 11G; SUGAR: 5G; PROTEIN: 53G

These grilled salmon skewers with yogurt sauce are tender, moist, and juicy with incredible flavor. A good source of heart-healthy omega-3 fatty acids, the salmon is served over a bed of fiber-, vitamin-, and mineral-rich romaine lettuce leaves. Light yet filling, this recipe is perfect for a hot summer day.

FOR THE SALMON SKEWERS

2 tablespoons rice vinegar

2 tablespoons olive oil,
    plus more for the grill

2 garlic cloves, minced

½ teaspoon dried dill

1½ pounds salmon fillet,
    cut into 1-inch squares

1 large lemon, thinly sliced

1 large lime, thinly sliced

FOR THE YOGURT SAUCE

3 garlic cloves, minced

⅛ teaspoon salt

1 tablespoon olive oil

1 cup nonfat plain yogurt

Chopped fresh parsley, for garnish

FOR THE SALAD

8 cups chopped romaine lettuce

1 tin flat anchovy fillets, drained

1 avocado, peeled and diced

1 cup croutons

2 lemons, halved

TO MAKE THE SALMON SKEWERS

1 Preheat a grill to medium heat, around 375°F.

2 In a medium bowl, stir together the rice vinegar, olive oil, garlic, and dill. Set aside.

3 Soak 8 (10-inch) wooden skewers in water for 30 minutes. Thread a skewer with a piece of salmon and 1 slice of lemon or lime folded in half. Repeat to fill all the skewers. Brush all sides of the salmon with the marinade.

4 Brush the grill grates with olive oil. Place the skewers on grill and cook for about 4 minutes per side, or until the salmon is cooked through and opaque. Alternatively, roast the skewers on a sheet pan in a 400°F oven for 12 to 15 minutes, until the salmon reaches an internal temperature of 145°F.

NUT
FREE

TO MAKE THE YOGURT SAUCE

1 Put the garlic in a small bowl and sprinkle it with the salt and 1½ teaspoons of olive oil. Mix well.

2 Stir in the yogurt to combine and drizzle the remaining 1½ teaspoons of olive oil on top.

3 Garnish with parsley and refrigerate until ready to use.

TO MAKE THE SALADS

1 Divide the romaine lettuce among 4 serving plates.

2 Remove the salmon skewers from the grill and place them on top of the lettuce.

3 Layer the plates with anchovies, avocado, and croutons, and top with the yogurt sauce. Serve each with a lemon half.

Sheet Pan Garlic-Baked Salmon and Asparagus

Serves 4 | Prep time: 5 minutes | Cook time: 15 minutes

➤ **PER SERVING** CALORIES: 224; TOTAL FAT: 10G; SATURATED FAT: 2G; TRANS FAT: 0G; CHOLESTEROL: 45MG; SODIUM: 78MG; TOTAL CARBOHYDRATE: 9G; FIBER: 4G; SUGAR: 2G; PROTEIN: 22G

This is a light, delicious, easy dish full of heart-healthy omega-3 fatty acids, high-quality protein, fiber, and vitamins and minerals. Salmon and asparagus are baked together for an effortlessly elegant meal.

Nonstick cooking spray

4 (4- to 6-ounce) boneless, skinless
   salmon fillets

1 pound asparagus,
   woody ends trimmed

2 tablespoons olive oil

2 tablespoons freshly squeezed
   lemon juice

2 garlic cloves, minced

1 lemon, sliced

Salt

Freshly ground black pepper

1 Preheat the oven to 350°F.

2 Spray a rimmed baking sheet with cooking spray.

3 Place the salmon and asparagus on the prepared sheet, spreading them out so nothing is crowded.

4 In a small bowl, whisk the olive oil, lemon juice, and garlic well. Drizzle over the salmon and asparagus. Layer lemon slices on top. Season with salt and pepper. Bake for 15 to 20 minutes until the salmon is opaque and the asparagus is soft. Serve immediately on its own, or alongside roasted potatoes, brown rice, or a green salad.

Did you know? Prebiotics are types of dietary fiber that feed the friendly bacteria in your gut. This helps the gut bacteria produce nutrients in your colon cells and leads to a healthier digestive system. Garlic and asparagus are two very good sources of prebiotics. Prebiotics should not be confused with probiotics, which are good bacteria in your intestines that keep your gut healthy.

5 MAIN INGREDIENTS	30 MINUTES OR FEWER	DAIRY FREE	LOW SODIUM	NUT FREE	

Roasted Salmon with Strawberry Arugula Salad

Serves 4 | Prep time: 15 minutes | Cook time: 15 minutes

➤ **PER SERVING** CALORIES: 310; TOTAL FAT: 18G; SATURATED FAT: 3G; TRANS FAT: 0G; CHOLESTEROL: 45MG; SODIUM: 140MG; TOTAL CARBOHYDRATE: 14G; FIBER: 5G; SUGAR: 5G; PROTEIN: 21G

Along with including two servings of fatty fish each week, consuming a couple servings of leafy greens each day can be one of the best habits to develop. Aside from their natural good taste and crunchy texture, eating greens and other raw vegetables each day boosts your intake of soluble fiber, which can reduce LDL (bad) cholesterol, as well as ensure you get adequate amounts of essential vitamins and minerals. With the added benefits of vitamin C- and fiber-rich strawberries, this dish is bursting with health-promoting nutrients.

4 (4- to 6-ounce) boneless, skinless salmon fillets

4 teaspoons plus 3 tablespoons olive oil, divided

Salt

Freshly ground black pepper

2 lemons, sliced

2 tablespoons balsamic vinegar

1 tablespoon Dijon mustard

2 garlic cloves, finely minced

2 cups sliced fresh strawberries

8 cups arugula, or fresh baby spinach

1 Preheat the oven to 450°F.

2 Line a rimmed sheet pan with parchment paper and place the salmon fillets on the sheet.

3 Drizzle each fillet with 1 teaspoon of olive oil and season with salt and pepper. Place 2 to 3 lemon slices on each fillet and bake for 10 to 12 minutes, depending on the thickness of the fillets, or until the salmon is opaque.

4 Meanwhile, in a small bowl, whisk the vinegar, Dijon mustard, remaining 3 tablespoons of olive oil, the garlic, a pinch of salt, and pepper. Refrigerate until ready to serve.

5 In a large bowl, toss together the strawberries and arugula. Divide the greens among 4 plates and drizzle with the dressing. Top each with a salmon fillet and serve.

	30 MINUTES OR FEWER	DAIRY FREE	LOW SODIUM	NUT FREE	

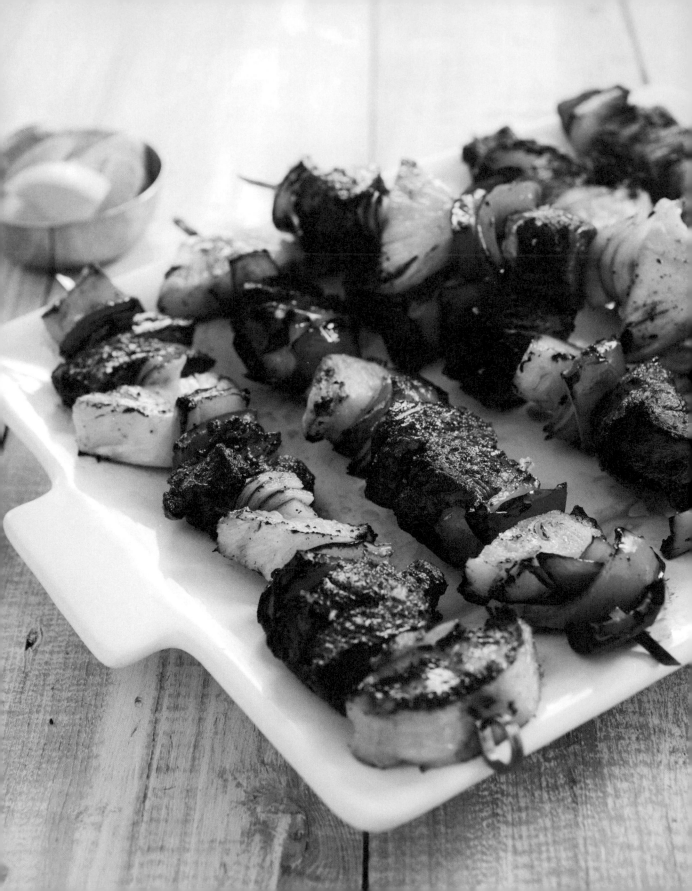

CHAPTER 8

Beef and Pork Mains

Italian Beef Tenderloin with White Beans

Serves 4 | Prep time: 10 minutes | Cook time: 15 minutes

➤ PER SERVING   CALORIES: 340; TOTAL FAT: 16G; SATURATED FAT: 6G; TRANS FAT: 0G; CHOLESTEROL: 95MG; SODIUM: 123MG; TOTAL CARBOHYDRATE: 11G; FIBER: 4G; SUGAR: 2G; PROTEIN: 35G

Current dietary recommendations are to limit the amount of red meat in the diet and to choose lean cuts that are low in fat. Beef can be part of a healthy diet; the trick is to start with lean cuts, then trim any fat from them. Of these cuts, one of the leanest is beef tenderloin. This recipe cooks the tenderloin quickly in a bit of olive oil, which helps preserve its tenderness. It also includes two fiber-, vitamin-, and mineral-rich ingredients—beans and spinach. With its intensely flavored sauce, this dish will leave you feeling energized, not weighed down.

1 tablespoon olive oil

4 (4-ounce) lean beef tenderloin filets, trimmed of fat

4 garlic cloves, chopped

Pinch red pepper flakes

6 cups fresh baby spinach

½ cup water

½ cup canned no-salt-added cannellini beans, drained and rinsed

1 cup chopped fresh tomatoes, with their juices

¼ cup chopped fresh basil leaves

Salt

Freshly ground black pepper

1 In a large skillet or sauté pan over medium-high heat, heat the olive oil until it shimmers.

2 Add the filets and cook for about 2 minutes, or until well browned on the bottom. Flip and cook for 2 minutes more, or until well browned on the other side. Transfer the filets to a plate and cover to keep warm.

3 Return the skillet to the heat and reduce the heat to medium. Add the garlic. Sauté for 20 to 30 seconds until golden brown.

4 Add the red pepper flakes and spinach. Cook for about 1 minute, stirring, until the spinach starts to wilt.

30 MINUTES OR FEWER	DAIRY FREE	LOW SODIUM	NUT FREE	ONE POT

5 Add the water, cover the skillet, and bring to a simmer. Cook for about 4 minutes until almost all the water evaporates.

6 Uncover the skillet and stir in the beans and the tomatoes with their juices. Cook for 1 minute, or until the sauce coats the spinach.

7 Add the filets back to the pan along with any collected juices on the plate, and add the basil. Cover the skillet and cook for 2 to 3 minutes for medium-rare to medium, or until your desired doneness.

8 Remove the beef and place one piece on each of 4 plates. Season the spinach and beans with salt and pepper, and spoon onto the plates with the beef.

Ingredient tip Remove the beef from the refrigerator 10 minutes before you cook so it will come to room temperature. The beef will cook more evenly and quickly this way.

Beef Tenderloin with Mustard and Herbs

Serves 4 | Prep time: 15 minutes | Cook time: 45 minutes

➤ **PER SERVING** CALORIES: 261; TOTAL FAT: 12G; SATURATED FAT: 5G; TRANS FAT: 0G; CHOLESTEROL: 95MG; SODIUM: 211MG; TOTAL CARBOHYDRATE: 3G; FIBER: 1G; SUGAR: 0G; PROTEIN: 31G

Beef is an excellent source of high-quality protein, iron, zinc, B vitamins, and other important minerals, but should be included sparingly in the diet. If red meat is something you would rather not give up, aim to keep portions in check, limit consumption to weekly, and don't make it the star of your plate. This recipe is low in fat, yet produces an elegant dish using a super easy herb crust. Serve alongside your favorite vegetables.

½ cup chopped fresh thyme leaves

½ cup chopped fresh oregano leaves

4 garlic cloves, finely chopped

Nonstick cooking spray

1 pound lean beef tenderloin, trimmed of fat

Freshly ground black pepper

Salt

3 tablespoons Dijon mustard

1 Preheat the oven to 400°F.

2 In a small bowl, mix together the thyme, oregano, and garlic. Set aside.

3 Spray the bottom of a roasting pan with cooking spray. Place the beef in the pan and season it with pepper and a pinch of salt. Evenly spread the Dijon mustard over the beef. Pat the herb mixture over the mustard. Insert an ovenproof meat thermometer into the beef so the tip is in the center of the thickest part. Bake uncovered for 35 to 45 minutes, or until the thermometer reads at least 140°F (for medium-rare).

4 Transfer the beef to a cutting board and cover it loosely with aluminum foil. Let stand for 15 minutes, or until the thermometer reads 145°F. The temperature will continue to rise about 5°F, and the beef will be easier to carve. Cut the beef into ½-inch-thick slices and serve.

Did you know? Meats and fish contain negligible amounts, if any, of carbohydrates or dietary fiber. Instead, they are protein and fat. Because of this, fill only one-fourth of your plate with meat, at least half your plate with high-fiber vegetables, and the remaining one-fourth with high-fiber grains. Alternatively, skip the grains and fill three-fourths of your plate with veggies.

5 MAIN INGREDIENTS	DAIRY FREE	LOW SODIUM	NUT FREE

Beef Tenderloin Steaks
with Balsamic Green Beans

Serves 4 | Prep time: 10 minutes | Cook time: 15 minutes

➤ **PER SERVING** CALORIES: 322; TOTAL FAT: 15G; SATURATED FAT: 6G; TRANS FAT: 0G; CHOLESTEROL: 95MG; SODIUM: 73MG; TOTAL CARBOHYDRATE: 13G; FIBER: 3G; SUGAR: 5G; PROTEIN: 33G

This appetizing recipe pairs simply seasoned beef tenderloin with a flavorful sauté of cholesterol-lowering foods, including onions, garlic, and high-fiber green beans. Quick to prepare, this outstanding meal is low in calories, nutrient rich, and easy enough to treat your family on a busy weeknight.

2 teaspoons olive oil

2 cups vertically sliced red onion

4 garlic cloves, minced

½ cup water

2 cups green beans, trimmed

2 tablespoons balsamic vinegar

4 (4-ounce) lean beef tenderloin steaks, trimmed of fat

Salt

Freshly ground black pepper

Nonstick cooking spray

1 In a medium saucepan over medium-high heat, heat the olive oil.

2 Add the red onion. Sauté for 6 minutes.

3 Add the garlic. Sauté for 1 minute.

4 Stir in the water. Cook for 4 minutes more, or until the onion is tender and most of the liquid has evaporated.

5 Add the green beans and vinegar. Cover the pan and cook for 4 minutes, or until the beans are crisp-tender. Remove from the heat and keep warm.

6 Season the steaks with a pinch of salt and pepper.

7 Heat a cast-iron skillet, or other heavy skillet, over medium-high heat. Coat the pan with cooking spray, add the steaks to the skillet, and cook for 3 minutes per side, or until your desired doneness. Let stand for 5 minutes. Serve the steaks with the green bean mixture.

30 MINUTES OR FEWER	DAIRY FREE	LOW SODIUM	NUT FREE

Veggie-Packed Open-Face Beef Burgers

Serves 4 | Prep time: 10 minutes | Cook time: 10 minutes

➤ **PER SERVING** CALORIES: 172; TOTAL FAT: 5G; SATURATED FAT: 2G; TRANS FAT: 0G; CHOLESTEROL: 49MG; SODIUM: 145MG; TOTAL CARBOHYDRATE: 9G; FIBER: 2G; SUGAR: 6G; PROTEIN: 19G

These produce-packed, open-face beef burgers are moist, juicy, and full of cholesterol-lowering fiber. Shredded apple and zucchini enhance the flavor of the burgers and keep this red meat dish on the healthy side. Serve open face on a bed of nutrient-rich greens with slices of fresh tomato, onion, and avocado, if you like.

12 ounces 90% lean ground beef

1 apple, shredded

1 medium zucchini, shredded

2 garlic cloves, minced

1 tablespoon ground mustard

Salt

Freshly ground black pepper

Nonstick cooking spray (optional)

1 In a large bowl, mix together the ground beef, apple, zucchini, garlic, mustard, and salt and pepper. Form the mixture into four (4-inch) patties.

2 Prepare a grill for medium heat, or preheat the broiler.

3 Cook the burgers for 6 to 8 minutes, flipping once halfway through the cooking time, until done to your liking. Alternatively, coat a large skillet with cooking spray and cook the burgers over medium heat for 6 to 8 minutes, flipping once. Serve with your favorite toppings.

Did you know? Eggs are not an essential ingredient for making beef burgers. The best burgers use only high-quality meat, seasonings, and optional veggie or fruit add-ins. Eggs are usually used in recipes that also use bread crumbs where they function to bind the bread with the meat.

	5 MAIN INGREDIENTS	30 MINUTES OR FEWER	DAIRY FREE	LOW SODIUM	NUT FREE	

Beef and Vegetable Kebabs

Serves 4 | Prep time: 15 minutes | Cook time: 5 minutes

➤ **PER SERVING** CALORIES: 342; TOTAL FAT: 16G; SATURATED FAT: 5G; TRANS FAT: 0G; CHOLESTEROL: 101MG; SODIUM: 79MG; TOTAL CARBOHYDRATE: 13G; FIBER: 3G; SUGAR: 7G; PROTEIN: 36G

These quick and easy steak kebabs are the perfect spring or summer meal, with their colorful mix of fiber-rich fruit and veggies. Lean sirloin keeps the saturated fat content in check, but be careful not to overcook these, as this cut of meat cooks quickly.

1 pound beef sirloin, cut into
   1-inch cubes

1 cup pineapple chunks

1 red bell pepper, cut into chunks

1 yellow bell pepper, cut into chunks

1 small yellow squash, sliced

1 large red onion, chopped

2 tablespoons olive oil

Salt

Freshly ground black pepper

1 Soak 8 (10-inch) wooden skewers in water for 30 minutes. Alternatively, use metal skewers (no soaking required!).

2 Preheat a grill to medium-high heat.

3 On a rimmed sheet pan, combine the beef cubes, pineapple, red and yellow bell peppers, squash, and red onion. Drizzle with the olive oil and toss until well coated. Season everything with salt and pepper. Skewer the meat, vegetables, and fruit alternately onto the skewers. Place the skewers on the grill and cook for about 5 minutes per side, rotating as needed until the meat, fruit, and vegetables are browned. Transfer to a large platter and serve.

5 MAIN INGREDIENTS	30 MINUTES OR FEWER	DAIRY FREE	LOW SODIUM	NUT FREE

Taco Lettuce Cups

Serves 4 | Prep time: 10 minutes | Cook time: 20 minutes

➤ **PER SERVING** CALORIES: 171; TOTAL FAT: 6G; SATURATED FAT: 2G; TRANS FAT: 0G; CHOLESTEROL: 65MG; SODIUM: 63MG; TOTAL CARBOHYDRATE: 6G; FIBER: 2G; SUGAR: 3G; PROTEIN: 25G

These lean ground beef lettuce wraps are delicious and light, and perfect for on-the-go nights. A healthier alternative to traditional tacos, a homemade mix of spices is used in place of packaged taco seasonings, which typically contain too much sodium, added sugars, and preservatives. To keep things light and calories in check, fiber-rich lettuce leaves are used in place of taco shells.

1½ teaspoons olive oil

2 garlic cloves, minced

1 small onion, minced

1 small bell pepper, any color, minced

1 pound 99% lean ground beef

1 teaspoon ground cumin

1 teaspoon chili powder

1 teaspoon paprika

¾ cup water

1 (4-ounce) can no-salt-added
tomato sauce

8 large romaine lettuce leaves,
washed and dried

Salt

Freshly ground black pepper

1 In a large skillet over medium heat, combine the olive oil, garlic, onion, and bell pepper. Sauté for about 3 minutes, until the onion is translucent.

2 Add the ground beef to the skillet. Cook for 7 to 10 minutes until no longer pink, or an internal temperature of 160°F, breaking the beef into smaller pieces with a spoon.

3 Add the cumin, chili powder, and paprika and mix well.

4 Stir in the water and tomato sauce. Reduce the heat to low and simmer the mixture for about 15 minutes.

5 Equally divide the meat among the lettuce leaves, placing it in the center of each leaf. Top with your favorite taco fixings.

Ingredient tip When purchasing lettuce, skip iceberg, which is very low in nutrition, and opt for healthier varieties, including romaine, red leaf, and butter lettuce. Research shows these three varieties contain significantly more antioxidants, vitamins, minerals, and fiber than iceberg lettuce.

	30 MINUTES OR FEWER	DAIRY FREE	LOW SODIUM	NUT FREE	ONE POT

Chili-Lime Beef and Black Bean Bowls

Serves 4 | Prep time: 10 minutes | Marinating time: 2 hours | Cook time: 10 minutes

➤ **PER SERVING** CALORIES: 439; TOTAL FAT: 13G; SATURATED FAT: 3G; TRANS FAT: 0G; CHOLESTEROL: 65MG; SODIUM: 99MG; TOTAL CARBOHYDRATE: 46G; FIBER: 11G; SUGAR: 2G; PROTEIN: 34G

This recipe embodies many of the healthy eating concepts you should strive for when making positive changes in your food choices: veggies, fiber, healthy fat, and lean protein. Super easy and simple to make ahead, these Mexican-inspired beef bowls can be made with virtually any lean cut of beef to create the perfect quick, delicious, nutrient-dense dinner.

¼ cup freshly squeezed lime juice
   (about 4 medium limes)

Salt

1 tablespoon chili powder

1 pound boneless thin beef sirloin
   tip steak (may be labeled as
   "for carne asada")

1 (15-ounce) can black beans,
   drained and rinsed

2 medium tomatoes, chopped

¼ cup chopped fresh cilantro, plus
   more for garnish (optional)

1 avocado, sliced

2 cups hot cooked brown rice

1 In a medium bowl, stir together the lime juice, a pinch of salt, and the chili powder. Set aside 1 teaspoon of the mixture in a separate bowl. Place half of the remaining mixture in a large resealable plastic bag. Add the beef, seal the bag, and shake to coat the meat. Refrigerate to marinate for at least 2 hours, or up to overnight.

2 In a medium bowl, combine the black beans, tomato, cilantro, and reserved lime juice–chili powder mixture. Toss together and refrigerator until ready to serve.

3 When ready to cook, heat a grill pan over medium-high heat.

4 Remove the meat from the bag and discard the marinade. Grill the beef for 2 to 3 minutes per side, or until your desired doneness. Remove from pan and let rest for 5 minutes. Slice into ¼-inch strips.

5 Divide the rice among 4 serving bowls. Top evenly with beans and beef. Layer with sliced avocado and additional cilantro, if desired.

DAIRY FREE	LOW SODIUM	NUT FREE

Spinach Salad with Grilled Pork Tenderloins and Nectarines

Serves 4 | Prep time: 5 minutes | Cook time: 10 minutes, plus 10 minutes resting

➤ **PER SERVING** CALORIES: 191; TOTAL FAT: 9G; SATURATED FAT: 2G; TRANS FAT: 0G; CHOLESTEROL: 26MG; SODIUM: 400MG; TOTAL CARBOHYDRATE: 15G; FIBER: 4G; SUGAR: 7G; PROTEIN: 13G

While marketing campaigns have dubbed pork "the other white meat" in an effort to compete with poultry, pork is still a red meat. However, many cuts of pork are as lean or leaner than chicken. Pork tenderloin, in particular, is just as lean as skinless chicken breast, so it can fit perfectly into your cholesterol-lowering diet. This delicious and nutritious recipe grills fresh nectarines with pork tenderloin and uses them to prepare a protein- and fiber-rich salad full of sweetness, crunch, and flavor.

8 ounces peppercorn-flavored pork tenderloin, trimmed of fat

Nonstick cooking spray

2 nectarines, or peaches, halved

2 (6-ounce) packages fresh baby spinach

2 tablespoons balsamic vinegar

2 tablespoons olive oil

1 cup sugar snap peas, strings removed

Freshly ground black pepper

1 Preheat the grill to medium-high heat.

2 Using a sharp knife, cut the pork horizontally through center of the meat, cutting to, but not through, the other side. Open the pork flat like a book.

3 Coat the grill rack with cooking spray. Place the pork and nectarine halves, cut-sides down, on the coated rack. Grill the pork for 5 minutes per side, or until an instant-read thermometer registers 160°F. Grill the nectarine halves for 4 to 5 minutes per side or until thoroughly heated. Remove the pork and nectarines from the grill. Let the pork rest for 10 minutes. Alternatively, cook under the broiler for about the same time and to the same internal temperature.

4 Cut the nectarine halves into slices. Thinly slice the pork.

5 In a large bowl, combine the spinach, vinegar, olive oil, and snap peas. Gently toss to coat.

6 Evenly divide the spinach mixture among 4 plates. Top each serving with nectarine and pork slices. Season with pepper, if desired.

5 MAIN INGREDIENTS	30 MINUTES OR FEWER	DAIRY FREE	LOW SODIUM	NUT FREE

Easy Cilantro Pork Stir-Fry

Serves 4 | Prep time: 15 minutes | Cook time: 10 minutes

➤ **PER SERVING** CALORIES: 236; TOTAL FAT: 14G; SATURATED FAT: 3G; TRANS FAT: 0G; CHOLESTEROL: 45MG; SODIUM: 37MG; TOTAL CARBOHYDRATE: 7G; FIBER: 2G; SUGAR: 2G; PROTEIN: 20G

This easy and nutritious stir-fry is made with just a handful of simple and natural ingredients. You won't miss the soy sauce in this dish, which is made with spicy fresh ginger and delicious fresh cilantro. Bell peppers are thinly sliced and stir-fried with the pork; however, you can substitute a medley of your favorite vegetables in their place.

4 garlic cloves, finely chopped, divided

1 tablespoon finely chopped peeled fresh ginger, divided

1 cup fresh cilantro leaves, or parsley leaves, chopped, divided

2 tablespoons plus 2 teaspoons olive oil, or peanut oil, divided

1 pound pork tenderloin, trimmed of fat and thinly sliced

2 red or green bell peppers, thinly sliced

1 tablespoon freshly squeezed lime juice (optional)

1 In a medium bowl, stir together half the garlic, 1½ teaspoons of ginger, ½ cup of cilantro, and 2 tablespoons of olive oil. Add the pork slices and toss to coat completely. Set aside for at least 10 minutes.

2 In a wok or large skillet over high heat, heat 1 teaspoon of olive oil until it shimmers.

3 Add the remaining garlic and 1½ teaspoons of ginger to the skillet and stir-fry for about 30 seconds, until they begin to brown.

4 Add the pork. Stir-fry for about 90 seconds, stirring constantly, until the pork changes color.

5 Add the bell peppers and continue to stir-fry for about 3 minutes more, until the peppers begin to soften.

6 Add the remaining ½ cup of cilantro and cook for 1 minute while tossing to blend the flavors.

7 Drizzle with lime juice (if using) and cook for 1 minute more. Serve immediately, either alone or with brown rice.

Substitution tip You can replace the peppers in this recipe with fresh onions, and, for vegetables, simply add 1 (16-ounce) bag frozen mixed stir-fry veggies in step 5, cooking for 8 to 10 minutes.

	5 MAIN INGREDIENTS	30 MINUTES OR FEWER	DAIRY FREE	LOW SODIUM	NUT FREE	

Pork Chops and Peppers

Serves 4 | Prep time: 10 minutes | Cook time: 15 minutes

➤ **PER SERVING** CALORIES: 259; TOTAL FAT: 17G; SATURATED FAT: 5G; TRANS FAT: 0G; CHOLESTEROL: 59MG; SODIUM: 44MG; TOTAL CARBOHYDRATE: 5G; FIBER: 1G; SUGAR: 2G; PROTEIN: 22G

Pork chops and peppers make a simple one-dish meal that is perfect for a busy weeknight. Because this recipe cooks quickly, lean cuts such as loin pork chops are the best choice. You can substitute your favorite vegetables in place of the peppers or simply add more veggies to boost the fiber, vitamin, and mineral content of this meal. Serve with brown rice, simmered canned black beans, or a seasonal fruit salad.

5 teaspoons olive oil, divided

4 (4-ounce, ¾-inch-thick) pork loin
   chops, trimmed of fat

Salt

Freshly ground black pepper

1 onion, chopped

4 garlic cloves, thinly sliced

2 bell peppers, any color, cut into strips

3 tablespoons red wine vinegar

Chopped fresh flat-leaf parsley,
   for garnish (optional)

1 In a large skillet over high heat, heat 1½ teaspoons of olive oil.

2 Season the pork with salt and pepper. Add to the skillet and cook for 3 minutes per side, or until cooked through (145°F on an instant-read thermometer). Remove from the pan and keep warm.

3 Return the skillet to the heat and reduce the heat to medium-high. Add the remaining 3½ teaspoons of olive oil, the onion, garlic, and bell peppers. Cook for 4 minutes, stirring occasionally, or until tender.

4 Increase the heat to high. Stir in the vinegar and cook for 1 minute, until the liquid reduces by half. Serve the pepper mixture with the pork, garnished with parsley (if using).

Ingredient tip Another way to increase the soluble fiber, vitamins, and minerals in your diet is to get into the habit of using beans as your side in place of starchy grains. Slow-digesting and filling, beans can aid in weight management.

5 MAIN INGREDIENTS	30 MINUTES OR FEWER	DAIRY FREE	LOW SODIUM	NUT FREE	ONE POT	

Pan-Roasted Pork Tenderloin and Eggplant

Serves 4 | Prep time: 5 minutes | Cook time: 35 minutes

➤ **PER SERVING** CALORIES: 332; TOTAL FAT: 17G; SATURATED FAT: 3G; TRANS FAT: 0G; CHOLESTEROL: 90MG; SODIUM: 67MG; TOTAL CARBOHYDRATE: 11G; FIBER: 4G; SUGAR: 5G; PROTEIN: 35G

This fragrant and flavorful pork tenderloin dish is seasoned with sweet cinnamon and fiery red pepper flakes for balance. Meaty eggplant accompanies the pork, absorbing flavors from the skillet until it is melt-in-your-mouth tender. High in protein, B vitamins, and fiber, this delicious dish comes together quickly and can be served with steamed brown rice, quinoa, or your favorite whole-grain pasta.

1 teaspoon ground cumin

1 teaspoon red pepper flakes

1 teaspoon cinnamon

Salt

4 garlic cloves, minced

1 pound pork tenderloin, trimmed of fat

2 tablespoons olive oil

1 medium eggplant (about 1½ pounds), cut into ½-inch cubes

½ cup apple cider vinegar

1 In a small bowl, stir together the cumin, red pepper flakes, and cinnamon. Add a pinch salt. Set aside.

2 Press the garlic evenly all over the pork.

3 In a large skillet over medium-high heat, heat the olive oil until it shimmers.

4 Place the garlic-rubbed pork in the skillet and sear on all 4 sides until it is a deep reddish-brown color, about 3 minutes per side. Transfer the browned pork to a plate.

5 Return the skillet to the heat and reduce the heat to medium.

6 Add the eggplant. Cook for 2 to 4 minutes, stirring until it absorbs some of the tenderloin flavors from the skillet and is tender. Sprinkle the spice blend over the eggplant and cook for about 1 minute, stirring to coat. ➤

DAIRY FREE	LOW SODIUM	NUT FREE	ONE POT

Pan-Roasted Pork Tenderloin and Eggplant

continued

7 Pour the vinegar into the skillet and stir, scraping up any browned bits from the bottom.

8 Return the pork to the skillet, spooning the eggplant over it. Cover the skillet and cook the pork without stirring for 10 to 12 minutes, until an instant-read thermometer inserted in the center registers 145°F to 150°F. Turn off the heat and let the pork rest, covered in the skillet, for 5 minutes. Transfer the pork to a cutting board and slice it into ½-inch-thick medallions. Arrange the pork slices on serving plates and spoon the eggplant over it.

Slow Cooker Honey Mustard Pork Roast

Serve 6 to 8 | Prep time: 10 minutes | Cook time: 6 to 7 hours on low heat,
or 3 to 4 hours on high heat

➤ **PER SERVING** CALORIES: 204; TOTAL FAT: 7G; SATURATED FAT: 3G; TRANS FAT: 0G; CHOLESTEROL: 80MG; SODIUM: 471MG; TOTAL CARBOHYDRATE: 6G; FIBER: 0G; SUGAR: 5G; PROTEIN: 26G

This simple low-fat, fiber- and protein-rich dish could easily be supplemented with some baby carrots, thickly sliced apple, halved Brussels sprouts, or a fresh green salad to complete the meal. The slow cooker is a great way to cook roasts, as the meat literally braises as it cooks, which makes it very tender and juicy.

Nonstick cooking spray

1 red onion, chopped

4 garlic cloves, minced

1 (2- to 3-pound) rolled boneless pork roast, trimmed of fat

¼ teaspoon freshly ground black pepper, plus more as needed

Salt

2 teaspoon dried basil, plus more as needed

¼ cup honey mustard, plus more as needed

¼ cup low-sodium chicken broth

¼ cup water (omit if not using cornstarch)

Cornstarch, for thickening (optional)

1 Spray a 4- to 6-quart slow cooker with cooking spray. Place the red onion and garlic in it.

2 Season the pork roast with the pepper, and salt to taste, and sprinkle with the basil.

3 Spread the honey mustard on the roast. Place the coated roast on top of the onion and garlic, and pour the chicken broth around the roast. Cover the cooker and cook for 6 to 7 hours on low heat or for 3 to 4 hours on high heat, or until an instant-read thermometer registers 145°F.

4 Remove the roast and cover with aluminum foil to keep warm while making the sauce.

5 In a medium saucepan over medium heat, combine the water, cornstarch (if using; whisk to combine with the water before adding the juices), and juices from the slow cooker, along with the cooked onion and garlic. Cook for 2 to 3 minutes until the mixture boils and thickens, stirring frequently. Taste and season with more pepper, basil, or honey mustard as needed.

6 Slice the roast and serve it with the sauce.

DAIRY FREE	LOW SODIUM	NUT FREE

Slow Cooker Stuffed Peppers with Pork

Serves 4 | Prep time: 10 minutes | Cook time: 6 hours on low heat, or 3 to 4 hours on high heat

➤ **PER SERVING** CALORIES: 371; TOTAL FAT: 21G; SATURATED FAT: 7G; TRANS FAT: 0G; CHOLESTEROL: 61MG; SODIUM: 74MG; TOTAL CARBOHYDRATE: 27G; FIBER: 7G; SUGAR: 10G; PROTEIN: 21G

With only five main ingredients, these hearty, fiber- and protein-rich stuffed peppers assemble in a snap. White beans are used in place of rice to boost the soluble fiber and vitamin and mineral content of this recipe, while adding a flavor boost and creamy texture. The use of a slow cooker cuts down the time you need to spend in the kitchen.

2 teaspoons olive oil

½ cup finely chopped onion

12 ounces 90% lean ground pork

1 cup canned white beans, drained and rinsed

4 medium green, red, and/or yellow bell peppers, tops trimmed off and discarded, ribbed and seeded

1 (15-ounce) can no-salt-added tomato sauce

Salt

Freshly ground black pepper

1 In a medium skillet over medium-high heat, heat the olive oil.

2 Add the onion. Cook for 3 minutes until softened, stirring occasionally. Remove from the heat and cool slightly.

3 In a large bowl, combine the ground pork, beans, and cooked onion. Mix to combine. Stuff each pepper with the pork mixture and arrange in the slow cooker.

4 Pour the tomato sauce over the peppers. Season with salt and pepper. Cover the cooker and cook for 6 hours on low heat or 3 to 4 hours on high heat. Serve hot with your favorite side of veggies.

Ingredient tip Line your slow cooker with a disposable slow cooker liner. Add the stuffed peppers as directed. Once your dish is finished cooking, remove the food from the cooker and simply discard the liner. *Do not lift or transport the disposable liner with food inside.*

5 MAIN INGREDIENTS	DAIRY FREE	LOW SODIUM	NUT FREE

Pork Tenderloin with Balsamic Onion-Fig Relish

Serves 4 | Prep time: 10 minutes | Cook time: 25 minutes

➤ **PER SERVING** CALORIES: 270; TOTAL FAT: 6G; SATURATED FAT: 2G; TRANS FAT: 0G; CHOLESTEROL: 45MG; SODIUM: 114MG; TOTAL CARBOHYDRATE: 36G; FIBER: 5G; SUGAR: 25G; PROTEIN: 21G

This delicious and easy pork tenderloin recipe tops the pork with a sweet and tangy balsamic onion and fig relish. It's simple to make with just a handful of ingredients, which is perfect for busy weeknights. Pork tenderloin is a lean source of high-quality protein, B vitamins, and iron, and the figs provide heart-healthy soluble fiber, as well as potassium, calcium, and magnesium. Serve this uniquely flavored dish with a side of steamed green beans.

1 (1-pound) pork tenderloin, trimmed of fat

Salt

Freshly ground black pepper

Nonstick cooking spray

10 dried Mission figs, coarsely chopped

3 tablespoons balsamic vinegar

2 tablespoons water

1½ teaspoons low-sodium soy sauce, or more balsamic vinegar

1 Vidalia onion, or yellow onion, chopped

1 Preheat the oven to 425°F.

2 Sprinkle the pork evenly with salt and pepper, and coat it with cooking spray.

3 Heat a medium ovenproof skillet or cast-iron pan over medium-high heat. Coat the skillet with cooking spray.

4 Add the pork. Cook for about 4 minutes per side, browning on all sides, turning occasionally.

5 While the pork browns, stir together the figs, vinegar, water, soy sauce, and onion in a small bowl.

6 When the pork is browned, remove the skillet from the heat. Add the fig-onion mixture and stir to loosen any browned bits from the bottom of the pan. Bake, uncovered, for 15 minutes, or until an instant-read thermometer registers 160°F.

7 Remove from the oven, stir the fig-onion mixture, cover the skillet loosely with aluminum foil, and let stand 5 minutes before slicing and serving.

	DAIRY FREE	LOW SODIUM	NUT FREE	

Spicy Pork Chops with Butternut Squash

Serves 4 | Prep time: 5 minutes | Cook time: 25 minutes

➤ PER SERVING   CALORIES: 283; TOTAL FAT: 11G; SATURATED FAT: 4G; TRANS FAT: 0G; CHOLESTEROL: 59MG; SODIUM: 88MG; TOTAL CARBOHYDRATE: 23G; FIBER: 7G; SUGAR: 6G; PROTEIN: 24G

This fragrantly spiced pork chop recipe incorporates creamy, delicious, and nutritious butternut squash to create a satisfying home-style dish. Butternut squash delivers an ample dose of dietary fiber, making it a heart-friendly choice. This colorful winter vegetable also provides significant amounts of the mineral potassium, which can balance dietary sodium and promote healthy blood pressure. Low in calories, fat, and sodium, this dish comes together quickly.

4 (4-ounce) boneless, center-cut loin pork chops (about ¾-inch thick), trimmed of fat
1 teaspoon pumpkin pie spice
½ teaspoon freshly ground black pepper, plus more for seasoning
Salt
Nonstick cooking spray
1 small butternut squash (about 1½ pounds)
1 cup chopped red onion
4 cups fresh baby spinach
¼ cup water

1 Sprinkle the pork evenly with the pumpkin pie spice, pepper, and a scant pinch of salt.

2 Heat a large nonstick skillet over medium-high heat. Coat it with cooking spray.

3 Add the pork to the skillet. Sauté for 3 to 4 minutes per side, or until cooked to an internal temperature of 145°F. Remove the pork from pan and keep warm.

4 While the pork cooks, pierce the squash several times with a fork. Place it on paper towels in the microwave and microwave on high power for 1 minute. Peel the squash and halve it lengthwise. Discard the seeds and membrane, then coarsely chop the flesh.

	30 MINUTES OR FEWER	DAIRY FREE	LOW SODIUM	NUT FREE	

5 Coat the skillet with a bit more cooking spray and place it over medium-high heat.

6 Add the squash. Cover the skillet and cook for 7 minutes, stirring occasionally.

7 Add the red onion. Cook, uncovered, for 5 minutes, stirring frequently.

8 Add the spinach and water. Cook for 2 to 3 minutes, uncovered, until the liquid evaporates, scraping the skillet's bottom to loosen any browned bits. Remove from the heat. Season with salt and pepper.

9 Spoon the squash mixture evenly over the pork to serve.

Ingredient tip Save some time with this recipe by purchasing precut butternut squash. Check the packaged vegetable area of your produce aisle for it. The cost of purchasing pre-cubed squash or buying a squash and preparing it yourself are comparable.

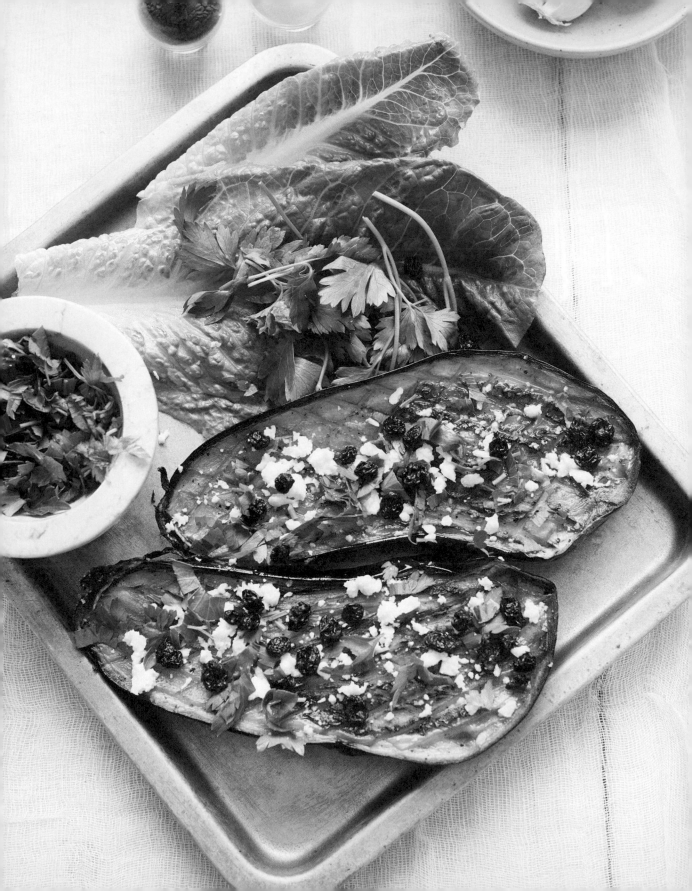

CHAPTER 9

Vegetables and Sides

Cauliflower and Broccoli Tots

Serves 4 | Prep time: 15 minutes | Cook time: 30 minutes

➤ **PER SERVING** CALORIES: 83; TOTAL FAT: 2G; SATURATED FAT: 0G; TRANS FAT: 0G; CHOLESTEROL: 47MG; SODIUM: 134MG; TOTAL CARBOHYDRATE: 13G; FIBER: 4G; SUGAR: 3G; PROTEIN: 5G

One way to increase your daily servings of fiber-rich veggies is to find creative recipes like this one, where ingredient swaps are made to make a comfort food more nutritious. These cauliflower and broccoli tots do just that by increasing the fiber, vitamins, and minerals and lowering the fat and calories of this side dish by swapping potatoes for veggies. These bites make a great snack or side dish.

2 slices whole-grain bread, torn into small pieces

2 cups mixed small cauliflower florets and chopped peeled stems

1 cup mixed small broccoli florets and chopped peeled stems

1 large egg

½ teaspoon paprika

Pinch salt (optional)

Freshly ground black pepper (optional)

Substitution tip Make these tots gluten-free by replacing the bread and water with 1 cup mashed potato, the amount you get from a peeled and boiled 10-ounce Russet potato.

1 Preheat the oven to 400°F.

2 Line a baking sheet with parchment paper.

3 In a small bowl, combine the bread with ½ cup water. Let soak for at least 15 minutes.

4 Meanwhile bring a medium pot filled two-thirds with water to a boil over high heat.

5 Add the cauliflower and broccoli and return the water to a boil. Boil for 1 minute. Immediately drain and cool the vegetables under cold running water. Drain well. Wrap the vegetables in a clean dishtowel or paper towels to remove as much moisture as possible.

6 In a food processor, combine the cooked vegetables, egg, paprika, and salt and pepper (if using).

7 Squeeze the bread very well to remove excess liquid and add it to the processor. Pulse just until the ingredients are chopped, but not puréed. Scoop the vegetable mixture by rounded tablespoons onto the prepared baking sheet. Dampen your fingers to prevent them from sticking and form the mixture into bite-sized cylinders. Bake for 20 to 25 minutes until browned and firm. Serve warm.

5 MAIN INGREDIENTS	BUDGET SAVER	DAIRY FREE	LOW SODIUM	NUT FREE

Mediterranean Orzo Salad

Serves 4 | Prep time: 5 minutes | Cook time: 10 minutes

➤ **PER SERVING** CALORIES: 339; TOTAL FAT: 5G; SATURATED FAT: 1G; TRANS FAT: 0G; CHOLESTEROL: 0MG; SODIUM: 58MG; TOTAL CARBOHYDRATE: 62G; FIBER: 11G; SUGAR: 4G; PROTEIN: 13G

This spinach and whole-wheat orzo salad is full of fiber, plant protein, and energy-boosting complex carbohydrates. With fresh tomatoes and creamy chickpeas, this salad is satisfying enough as a light main course, or perfect to serve alongside grilled mains.

8 ounces whole-wheat orzo (rice-shaped pasta)

4 cups packed fresh baby spinach

1 cup cherry tomatoes, halved

1 (15-ounce) can chickpeas, drained and rinsed

¼ cup chopped fresh basil leaves

1 tablespoon olive oil

1 In a large pot of boiling water over high heat, cook the orzo for 8 to 10 minutes until al dente. Drain, rinse under cold running water, and drain again. Transfer to a large bowl.

2 Add the spinach, tomatoes, chickpeas, basil, and olive oil. Toss to combine and serve.

5 MAIN INGREDIENTS	30 MINUTES OR FEWER	BUDGET SAVER	DAIRY FREE	LOW SODIUM	NUT FREE

Eggplant Topped with Raisins and Feta

Serves 2 | Prep time: 10 minutes | Cook time: 15 minutes

➤ **PER SERVING** CALORIES: 384; TOTAL FAT: 32G; SATURATED FAT: 6G; TRANS FAT: 0G; CHOLESTEROL: 13MG; SODIUM: 174MG; TOTAL CARBOHYDRATE: 27G; FIBER: 7G; SUGAR: 16G; PROTEIN: 5G

Eggplant is a culinary chameleon, absorbing herbs and spices to become any number of dishes. This recipe dresses the eggplant simply with garlic, vinegar, and olive oil, which is then grilled and topped with a sprinkling of raisins, feta cheese, and fresh parsley. Full of flavor with a satisfying meaty texture, this side dish works well with grilled fish or poultry.

¼ cup feta cheese

1 tablespoon finely chopped
   fresh parsley leaves

¼ cup olive oil

2 tablespoons balsamic vinegar

Salt

1 medium eggplant (about
   1½ pounds), trimmed
   and halved lengthwise

2 tablespoons raisins

Freshly ground black pepper

1 In a small bowl, combine the feta and parsley.

2 In another small bowl, whisk the olive oil, vinegar, and a pinch of salt.

3 Preheat a grill to medium-high heat, and line the grill rack with foil, if needed.

4 Brush the eggplant halves with the marinade and season with salt and pepper. Reserve any remaining marinade. Place the eggplant to the grill, cut-side down. Close the cover and cook for 5 to 7 minutes per side, turning once halfway through the cooking time, until the eggplant is very tender and lightly charred. Alternatively, roast the eggplant in a 400°F oven for 20 to 25 minutes.

5 Remove from the grill and top each half with the feta mixture and a sprinkle of raisins. Drizzle with the reserved marinade and serve.

5 MAIN INGREDIENTS	30 MINUTES OR FEWER	BUDGET SAVER	LOW SODIUM	NUT FREE

Parmesan-Crusted Summer Squash

Serves 6 | Prep time: 10 minutes | Cook time: 25 minutes

➤ **PER SERVING** CALORIES: 100; TOTAL FAT: 3G; SATURATED FAT: 2G; TRANS FAT: 0G; CHOLESTEROL: 38MG; SODIUM: 171MG; TOTAL CARBOHYDRATE: 11G; FIBER: 3G; SUGAR: 3G; PROTEIN: 7G

These baked Parmesan-crusted summer squash are a healthy alternative to fried side dishes like French fries. Perfectly seasoned with a delicious herb mix, this easy side dish is high in dietary fiber, protein, and heart-healthy B vitamins and minerals. Serve these with your favorite lean meat, fish, or plant-based protein.

2 large egg whites, beaten

1 large egg

½ cup whole-wheat panko bread crumbs

½ cup shredded Parmesan cheese

¼ cup chopped fresh parsley leaves

2 pounds zucchini, or yellow squash, cut on an angle into ½-inch-thick rounds

Freshly ground black pepper

1 Preheat the oven to 425°F.

2 Line a baking sheet with parchment paper and set aside.

3 In a small shallow bowl, whisk the egg whites and egg. Set aside.

4 In another shallow bowl, combine the bread crumbs, Parmesan cheese, and parsley. Set aside.

5 Dip the zucchini rounds into the eggs and into the bread crumb mixture. Place them on the prepared sheet. Bake for 20 to 25 minutes, until golden brown and crisp. Serve hot seasoned with pepper.

Ingredient tip For a variation, replace the eggs with ½ cup of your favorite prepared pesto. Spread a bit on both sides of the rounds, then press gently to coat both sides with the bread crumb mixture.

5 MAIN INGREDIENTS	BUDGET SAVER	DAIRY FREE	LOW SODIUM	NUT FREE

Easy Roasted Asparagus

Serves 4 | Prep time: 5 minutes | Cook time: 15 minutes

➤ **PER SERVING** CALORIES: 82; TOTAL FAT: 4G; SATURATED FAT: 1G; TRANS FAT: 0G; CHOLESTEROL: 0MG; SODIUM: 5MG; TOTAL CARBOHYDRATE: 10G; FIBER: 5G; SUGAR: 4G; PROTEIN: 5G

If you avoid adding asparagus to your plate, you might be harboring some unpleasant memories of a heavily boiled version of this vegetable. Forget those images and prepare your taste buds for a delicious experience. Roasting asparagus gives the tips a salty crunch and makes the stems melt-in-your-mouth tender. A good source of fiber, heart-healthy potassium, and folate and a natural diuretic, take advantage of this springtime vegetable when it is in season.

2 pounds asparagus, woody ends removed

1 tablespoon olive oil

Salt

Freshly ground black pepper

1 Preheat the oven to 450°F.

2 Line two baking sheets with aluminum foil for easier cleanup, if desired.

3 Spread the asparagus on the prepared sheets. Drizzle the olive oil evenly over the top and use your fingers to gently rub each stalk with the olive oil. Season with salt and pepper. Roast for 12 to 15 minutes. You will know the asparagus is done when it turns bright green, the stems are tender, and the tips begin to get crisp. Serve hot.

Ingredient tip Thicker, larger asparagus stalks work best for roasting. Cooking time will vary based on the thickness—small or very thin stalks may take 10 minutes or less to roast.

5 MAIN INGREDIENTS	30 MINUTES OR FEWER	BUDGET SAVER	DAIRY FREE	LOW SODIUM	NUT FREE	ONE POT	

Caramelized Root Vegetables

Serves 4 | Prep time: 10 minutes | Cook time: 35 minutes

➤ **PER SERVING** CALORIES: 108; TOTAL FAT: 4G; SATURATED FAT: 1G; TRANS FAT: 0G; CHOLESTEROL: 0MG; SODIUM: 37MG; TOTAL CARBOHYDRATE: 18G; FIBER: 4G; SUGAR: 6G; PROTEIN: 2G

Roasted root vegetables are a great source of fiber-rich complex carbohydrates, and they are packed with antioxidants, essential vitamins, and minerals. The roasting process caramelizes the natural sugar of the vegetables so, after roasting, they taste amazingly sweet and delicious and are a perfect cure for a sweet craving. Feel free to experiment with your favorite root vegetables.

1 medium sweet potato, chopped into chunks

1 cup (¾-inch) peeled carrot chunks

1 cup (¾-inch) peeled parsnip chunks

1 medium red onion, cut into ½-inch wedges

1 tablespoon olive oil

1 tablespoon fresh oregano leaves, chopped

Salt

Freshly ground black pepper

1 Preheat the oven to 375°F.

2 Line a rimmed baking sheet with parchment paper and set aside.

3 In a large microwave-safe dish, combine the sweet potato, carrots, parsnip, and red onion. Add ½ inch of water, cover loosely, and microwave on high power for 4 minutes. Drain.

4 Add the olive oil and oregano, season with salt and pepper, and toss to coat. Spread the vegetables on the prepared sheet. Roast for 35 minutes, until the vegetables are caramelized and tender. Remove from the oven halfway through the cooking time to turn and toss the veggies. Serve hot.

Ingredient tip Microwaving the vegetables for a few minutes before roasting cuts down on cooking time. You can skip this step if you have the time and simply increase the roasting time to about 50 minutes.

5 MAIN INGREDIENTS	DAIRY FREE	LOW SODIUM	NUT FREE

Cauliflower Mashed "Potatoes"

Serves 4 | Prep time: 10 minutes | Cook time: 10 minutes

➤ **PER SERVING** CALORIES: 70; TOTAL FAT: 4G; SATURATED FAT: 1G; TRANS FAT: 0G; CHOLESTEROL: 0MG;
SODIUM: 44MG; TOTAL CARBOHYDRATE: 9G; FIBER: 4G; SUGAR: 3G; PROTEIN: 3G

This recipe is a creamy, delicious, gluten-free, low-carb, and vegan alternative to mashed potatoes. Cauliflower is a cruciferous vegetable and an excellent source of the antioxidant vitamin C, and a very good source of dietary fiber, B vitamins, minerals, and plant-based omega-3 fatty acids. You won't miss the potatoes in this recipe, which makes a perfect side dish for meats, fish, and plant-based meals.

1 large head cauliflower (about
   3 pounds), trimmed and cut
   into florets

4 garlic cloves, peeled

1 tablespoon olive oil, plus more
   for garnish (optional)

Pinch salt

Freshly ground black pepper

Chopped fresh chives, for garnish
   (optional)

Chopped fresh thyme leaves,
   for garnish (optional)

1 Bring a large pot of salted water to a boil over high heat. Add the cauliflower and garlic. Cook for about 10 minutes, or until the cauliflower is fork-tender. Drain, reserving ¼ cup of the cooking liquid. Return the cauliflower to the hot pan. Let stand, covered and off the heat, for 2 to 3 minutes.

2 Transfer the cauliflower, garlic, and reserved cooking liquid to a food processor. Add the olive oil, salt, and pepper to taste. Purée until smooth. Transfer to a serving bowl and garnish with a drizzle of olive oil, chives, or thyme (if using). Serve immediately.

Substitution tip Save time by buying riced cauliflower from the produce section of your grocery store. Two (16-ounce) packages are roughly equivalent to 1 large head of cauliflower (about 3 pounds).

5 MAIN INGREDIENTS	30 MINUTES OR FEWER	BUDGET SAVER	DAIRY FREE	LOW SODIUM	NUT FREE

Baked Sweet Potato Fries

Serves 4 | Prep time: 10 minutes | Cook time: 30 minutes

➤ **PER SERVING** CALORIES: 200; TOTAL FAT: 8G; SATURATED FAT: 1G; TRANS FAT: 0G; CHOLESTEROL: 0MG; SODIUM: 17MG; TOTAL CARBOHYDRATE: 32G; FIBER: 4G; SUGAR: 6G; PROTEIN: 2G

Oven-baked sweet potato fries are super easy to make, extremely nutritious, and rather addictive. One sweet potato contains more than twice the amount of vitamin A you need for the day (in the form of beta-carotene), and is a very good source of vitamin C as well as dietary fiber, potassium, and B vitamins. Tossed with olive oil and lightly seasoned, these sweet potato fries are a healthy side dish or snack.

2 tablespoons olive oil

2 teaspoons paprika

1 teaspoon garlic powder

½ teaspoon ground cumin (optional)

¼ teaspoon cayenne pepper (optional)

Salt

Freshly ground black pepper

2 pounds orange-fleshed sweet potatoes (about 1 medium per person), rinsed, dried, and cut into 1-inch wedges

1 Preheat the oven to 450°F.

2 Line a rimmed baking sheet with parchment paper.

3 In a large bowl, stir together the olive oil, paprika, garlic powder, and cumin and cayenne (if using). Season with salt and pepper.

4 Add the sweet potatoes and toss until they are evenly coated. Transfer to the prepared sheet and spread the sweet potatoes into a single layer. Try not to overcrowd them or have multiple layers of fries—you want them roasted, not steamed. Bake for 25 to 30 minutes, turning the fries once or twice, so they cook evenly.

5 Remove from the oven once the edges begin to brown slightly, and the fries begin to crisp. Serve hot.

	5 MAIN INGREDIENTS	BUDGET SAVER	DAIRY FREE	LOW SODIUM	NUT FREE	

Broccoli Slaw

Serves 4 | Prep time: 10 minutes

➤ **PER SERVING** CALORIES: 258; TOTAL FAT: 23G; SATURATED FAT: 3G; TRANS FAT: 0G; CHOLESTEROL: 0MG; SODIUM: 27MG; TOTAL CARBOHYDRATE: 11G; FIBER: 4G; SUGAR: 4G; PROTEIN: 6G

Broccoli slaw is a healthy side dish and wonderful alternative to the typical cabbage variety. It is low in calories and high in vitamins A and C, and has an impressive fiber content. Incredibly versatile, it's equally tasty in raw or cooked form, with either a sweet or a savory kick. This slaw is tossed in a tangy dressing and comes together in just minutes.

1 (12-ounce) package broccoli coleslaw

½ cup diced sweet Vidalia onion

¼ cup olive oil

¼ cup apple cider vinegar

1 teaspoon dill weed

¼ teaspoon freshly ground black pepper

Salt

½ cup sliced almonds

1 In a large bowl, mix together the broccoli slaw and onion. Set aside.

2 In a small bowl, whisk the olive oil, vinegar, dill, pepper, and salt to taste. Pour the dressing over the coleslaw and stir to coat.

3 Just before serving, mix in the almonds.

Ingredient tip Broccoli coleslaw is prewashed, pre-shredded, and premixed, making it a convenient way to add fiber and nutrient-rich veggies to your diet. Plus, you can steam or microwave it right in the bag. Just snip a corner to vent, and microwave on high power for 3 to 3½ minutes.

5 MAIN INGREDIENTS	30 MINUTES OR FEWER	BUDGET SAVER	DAIRY FREE	LOW SODIUM	

Parsnip Fries

Serves 4 | Prep time: 5 minutes | Cook time: 25 minutes

➤ **PER SERVING** CALORIES: 224; TOTAL FAT: 8G; SATURATED FAT: 1G; TRANS FAT: 0G; CHOLESTEROL: 0MG; SODIUM: 23MG; TOTAL CARBOHYDRATE: 39G; FIBER: 8G; SUGAR: 11G; PROTEIN: 3G

Parsnips are a root vegetable closely related to the carrot, and their long shelf life and low cost make them an economical addition to your diet. High in dietary fiber, folate, potassium, and vitamin C, roasting parsnips enhances their unique flavor and creates a much healthier alternative to traditional French fries.

2 pounds parsnips, peeled, cut into 3-by-½-inch strips

2 garlic cloves, minced

1 tablespoon finely chopped fresh rosemary leaves

2 tablespoons olive oil

Salt

Freshly ground black pepper

1 Preheat the oven to 450°F.

2 On a large rimmed baking sheet, mix together the parsnips, garlic, rosemary, and olive oil. Season with salt and pepper and toss to coat. Spread the parsnips in a single layer.

3 Roast for 10 minutes. Turn the parsnips and roast for 10 to 15 minutes longer until tender and browned in spots. Serve hot.

5 MAIN INGREDIENTS	30 MINUTES OR FEWER	BUDGET SAVER	DAIRY FREE	LOW SODIUM	NUT FREE	ONE POT	

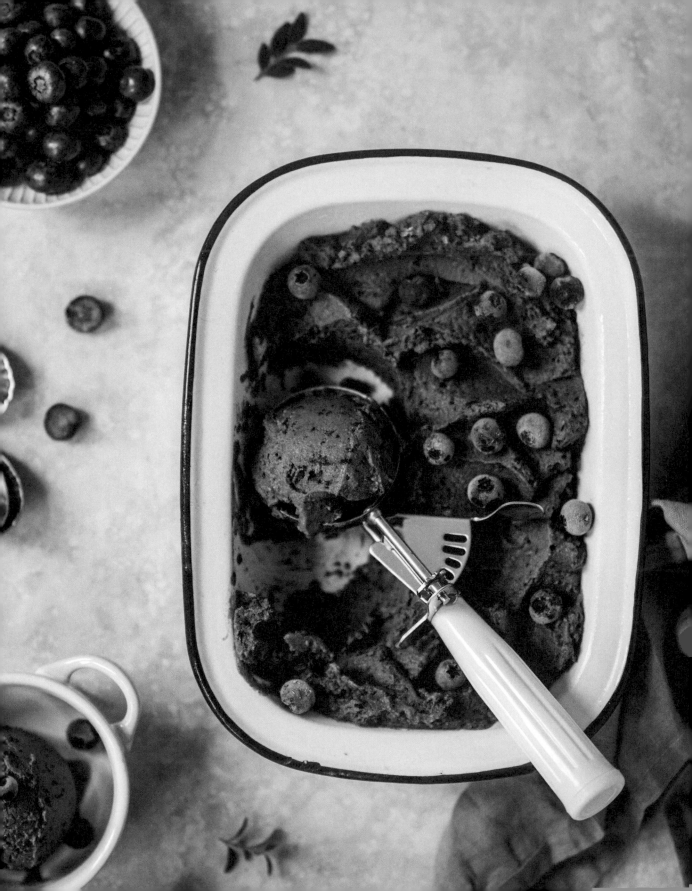

Desserts

DIY Strawberry Ice Cream

Serves 4 | Prep time: 10 minutes | Chill time: 2 to 3 hours

➤ **PER SERVING** CALORIES: 126; TOTAL FAT: 11G; SATURATED FAT: 9G; TRANS FAT: 0G; CHOLESTEROL: 0MG; SODIUM: 16MG; TOTAL CARBOHYDRATE: 7G; FIBER: 1G; SUGAR: 3G; PROTEIN: 1G

This dairy-free vegan strawberry ice cream tastes just like soft serve, but it's much healthier because it contains no added sugars, heavy cream, fillers, or preservatives. No ice cream maker is needed, and the strawberries, this ice cream's main ingredient, are incredibly high in beneficial antioxidants, vitamin C, and dietary fiber with their own natural sweetness.

8 ounces frozen strawberries

8 ounces coconut milk (not coconut cream)

1 teaspoon freshly squeezed lemon juice

⅛ teaspoon liquid stevia

1 In a high-speed blender or food processor, combine the strawberries, coconut milk, lemon juice, and stevia. Process just until smooth. Transfer to a lidded plastic container and freeze for 30 minutes.

2 With a sturdy whisk or fork, churn the mixture, breaking up any ice crystals or frozen bits. Return it to the freezer for 30 minutes more. Repeat churning and freezing until it firms up (2 to 3 hours total). Enjoy.

Ingredient tip Regular full-fat coconut milk produces the creamiest ice cream, but you can opt for light coconut milk, which is lower in calories and saturated fat. You can also replace the stevia with ¼ cup agave, pure maple syrup, or honey, but this will increase the calorie count.

	5 MAIN INGREDIENTS	BUDGET SAVER	DAIRY FREE	LOW SODIUM	NUT FREE	

Blueberry Blender Nice Cream

Serves 2 | Prep time: 5 minutes

➤ **PER SERVING** CALORIES: 198; TOTAL FAT: 1G; SATURATED FAT: 0G; TRANS FAT: 0G; CHOLESTEROL: 0MG; SODIUM: 3MG; TOTAL CARBOHYDRATE: 50G; FIBER: 7G; SUGAR: 28G; PROTEIN: 2G

This recipe is about as simple and healthy as it gets. All you need are some frozen bananas and antioxidant-rich blueberries to make a deliciously sweet, dairy-free, frozen dessert. Blueberries are highly nutritious and including them in your diet has been shown to protect against heart disease and promote healthy blood pressure. Combined with potassium-rich bananas, this guilt-free, delicious dessert is high in fiber, B vitamins, minerals, and disease-protective phytonutrients.

3 ripe bananas, sliced and frozen

1 cup frozen blueberries

Vanilla extract, to add (optional)

Hemp seeds, to add (optional)

Nut butter, to add (optional)

Ground cinnamon, to add (optional)

Cacao nibs or powder, to add (optional)

Fresh blueberries, for garnish (optional)

In a high-speed blender or food processor, combine the bananas and blueberries, along with any add-ins, as desired. Blend for about 5 minutes until smooth and creamy. Serve immediately topped with fresh blueberries (if using).

5 MAIN INGREDIENTS	30 MINUTES OR FEWER	BUDGET SAVER	DAIRY FREE	LOW SODIUM	NUT FREE	ONE POT

Peppermint Mocha

Serves 4 | Prep time: 5 minutes | Cook time: 5 minutes

➤ **PER SERVING** CALORIES: 70; TOTAL FAT: 3G; SATURATED FAT: 2G; TRANS FAT: 0G; CHOLESTEROL: 2MG; SODIUM: 16MG; TOTAL CARBOHYDRATE: 11G; FIBER: 1G; SUGAR: 9G; PROTEIN: 2G

Full of festive flavor, coffee shop style peppermint mocha drinks are a staple in the diet of many mocha-holics. Unfortunately, this coffee shop holiday favorite is high in calories, fat, added sugars, and fillers, including imitation vanilla and soy lecithin. The good news is, you can whip up your own skinny peppermint mocha latte at home in just a few minutes, and create a healthier alternative that boasts minty flavor while saving you calories, fat, and sugar.

2 cups strong-brewed coffee

½ cup 1% milk, divided

2½ tablespoons sugar

1 tablespoon unsweetened
  cocoa powder

1 ounce 60% bittersweet chocolate,
  finely chopped

1 or 2 drops food-grade peppermint oil

1 In a small saucepan over low heat, combine the coffee and ¼ cup of milk.

2 Stir in the sugar, cocoa powder, and chocolate. Cook for 4 minutes, or until the chocolate melts, stirring frequently (do not simmer).

3 Stir in the peppermint oil. Divide the hot coffee mixture among 4 mugs.

4 Place the remaining ¼ cup of milk in a microwave-safe 1-cup container with a lid. Cover and shake vigorously for 1 minute, of until the milk is frothy and doubled in volume. Remove the lid. Microwave on high power for 30 seconds. Top each coffee cup with a dollop of milk froth. Divide any remaining hot milk evenly among the cups.

Ingredient tip Peppermint oil, much more concentrated than alcohol-diluted extract, lends bold mint flavor with just a couple drops. While very dark chocolate is highest in anti-oxidants, bittersweet works best here, making for a rounder, smoother flavor.

	30 MINUTES OR FEWER	BUDGET SAVER	LOW SODIUM	NUT FREE	ONE POT	

Flourless Chocolate Cookies

Makes 9 cookies | Prep time: 5 minutes | Cook time: 10 minutes

➤ **PER SERVING (1 COOKIE)** CALORIES: 196; TOTAL FAT: 14G; SATURATED FAT: 1G; TRANS FAT: 0G; CHOLESTEROL: 0MG; SODIUM: 14MG; TOTAL CARBOHYDRATE: 16G; FIBER: 4G; SUGAR: 11G; PROTEIN: 5G

These flourless chocolate cookies are made with just four ingredients and are vegan, gluten-free, and grain-free. Nut butters are a good source of heart-healthy fats and plant-based protein, and cacao is high in beneficial antioxidants. You could also make these cookies nut-free by substituting sunflower butter in place of the almond butter. These cookies take just minutes to prepare and the results are delicious.

1 cup almond butter, or your favorite nut or seed butter

¼ cup plus 1 tablespoon honey, or pure maple syrup

2 tablespoons unsweetened cocoa powder, or cacao powder

¼ teaspoon baking powder

Shredded coconut, to add (optional)

Dried cherries, to add (optional)

Semisweet chocolate chips, to add (optional)

1 Preheat the oven to 350°F.

2 Line a baking sheet with parchment paper and set aside.

3 In a food processor, combine the almond butter, honey, cocoa powder, baking powder, and any add-ins, as desired. Process until combined. Divide the mixture into 9 portions, and form each into a ball. Place the balls on the prepared sheet. Bake for 10 minutes.

4 Let cool completely before removing from the baking sheet or the cookies will crumble.

5 Enjoy immediately or refrigerate in an airtight container for about 1 week.

Ingredient tip For fast prep and even portions, use a cookie scoop to form the balls.

5 MAIN INGREDIENTS	30 MINUTES OR FEWER	BUDGET SAVER	DAIRY FREE	LOW SODIUM	ONE POT

No-Bake Cookie Dough Bites

Makes 12 cookie bites | Prep time: 10 minutes | Chill time: 10 minutes

➤ **PER SERVING (1 COOKIE BITE)** CALORIES: 134; TOTAL FAT: 5G; SATURATED FAT: 0G; TRANS FAT: 0G; CHOLESTEROL: 0MG; SODIUM: 0MG; TOTAL CARBOHYDRATE: 20G; FIBER: 3G; SUGAR: 14G; PROTEIN: 3G

These no-bake cookie dough bites are full of cholesterol-lowering ingredients and have no dairy, eggs, or refined sugars. Soluble fiber–rich old-fashioned rolled oats are processed with heart-healthy almonds and fiber-, vitamin-, and mineral-rich dates to create delicious, moist cookie dough bites. Enjoy one of these with a cold glass of your favorite dairy or plant-based milk.

1 cup raw, unsalted whole almonds

1 cup old-fashioned rolled oats

10 pitted Medjool dates

¼ cup water

Pinch cinnamon (optional)

Cacao nibs, to add (optional)

Semisweet chocolate chips,
   to add (optional)

1 Line a baking sheet with parchment paper and set aside.

2 In a food processor, combine the almonds and oats. Process into a fine powder.

3 Add the dates and continue to process.

4 Add the water, a little at a time (you may not need it all), until a pastelike dough forms. Roll the dough into 12 little balls (about 1 tablespoon each), or use a cookie scoop to scoop the batter. Place the balls onto the prepared sheet. Refrigerate for about 10 minutes until the dough firms up a bit. Enjoy!

Did you know? Medjool dates, commonly referred to as the king of dates, are high in fiber, potassium, magnesium, calcium, iron, and B vitamins. Satisfyingly chewy and flavorful, they can take the place of sugar in recipes such as this, or in smoothies, and are a wonderful snack all by themselves.

	5 MAIN INGREDIENTS	30 MINUTES OR FEWER	BUDGET SAVER	DAIRY FREE	LOW SODIUM	ONE POT	

Banana Bread Cookies

Makes 12 cookies | Prep time: 5 minutes | Cook time: 12 minutes

➤ **PER SERVING (1 COOKIE)** CALORIES: 76; TOTAL FAT: 3G; SATURATED FAT: 1G; TRANS FAT: 0G; CHOLESTEROL: 0MG; SODIUM: 1MG; TOTAL CARBOHYDRATE: 11G; FIBER: 2G; SUGAR: 3G; PROTEIN: 2G

These soft and chewy cookies taste just like banana bread, but they have no added sugars, dairy, or eggs, and are naturally gluten-free. Made with soluble fiber–rich oat bran and bananas, and heart-healthy nut butter, all you need is one bowl and less than 20 minutes to whip up these easy, nutritious cookies.

2 large overripe bananas, mashed

1 cup oat bran, plus more as needed

¼ cup cashew butter, or your favorite nut or seed butter

1 Preheat the oven to 350°F.

2 Line a baking sheet with parchment paper and set aside.

3 In a large bowl, mix together the bananas, oat bran, and cashew butter. If the batter is too thin, add more oat bran. Using your hands or a cookie scoop, form the batter into 12 balls and place them on the prepared sheet. Press each ball into a cookie shape. Bake for 12 minutes, or until slightly firm on the edges.

4 Remove from the oven and let cool for 5 minutes before enjoying.

Ingredient tip Many three-ingredient banana bread cookie recipes call for old-fashioned rolled oats. However, the use of oat bran here gives them a more breadlike texture. Feel free to use what you prefer.

5 MAIN INGREDIENTS	30 MINUTES OR FEWER	BUDGET SAVER	DAIRY FREE	LOW SODIUM

Pumpkin Cake Pops

Makes 12 cake pops | Prep time: 5 minutes | Cook time: 15 minutes

➤ **PER SERVING (1 CAKE POP)** CALORIES: 61; TOTAL FAT: 1G; SATURATED FAT: 0G; TRANS FAT: 0G; CHOLESTEROL: 0MG; SODIUM: 1MG; TOTAL CARBOHYDRATE: 12G; FIBER: 5G; SUGAR: 5G; PROTEIN: 2G

These healthy, three-ingredient cake pops are soft and cakelike and take only minutes to prepare. Naturally vegan and gluten-free, this pleasantly sweet dessert is also low in fat and added sugars. Canned 100% pure pumpkin is mixed with fiber-rich coconut flour and a dash of sugar to create a nutritious dessert or snack that can satisfy your sweet tooth while adding vitamin A and fiber to your diet.

Nonstick cooking spray

1 cup coconut flour, sifted

¾ cup 100% pumpkin (not pumpkin pie filling)

¼ cup granulated sweetener of choice

1 teaspoon pumpkin pie spice (optional)

Semisweet chocolate chips, to add (optional)

1 Preheat the oven to 350°F.

2 Spray a large baking sheet with cooking spray and set aside.

3 In a large bowl, stir together the coconut flour, pumpkin, sweetener, and pumpkin pie spice (if using).

4 Add the chocolate chips (if using), and mix until fully incorporated.

5 Using your hands, shape the dough into 12 small balls and place them on the prepared sheet. Depending on the texture you want, bake for about 10 minutes (for a softer cake texture) to 15 minutes (for a very dense and crumbly texture).

6 Remove from oven and let cool completely before eating.

Substitution tip Coconut flour is used in this recipe because this type of flour naturally has a cakelike texture. Coconut flour is low in fat and very low in dietary fiber, making it a good fit for a cholesterol-lowering diet. However, you can substitute oat flour for a denser product or use regular cake flour.

5 MAIN INGREDIENTS	30 MINUTES OR FEWER	BUDGET SAVER	DAIRY FREE	LOW SODIUM	NUT FREE

Spiced Baked Apples

Serves 4 | Prep time: 10 minutes | Cook time: 40 minutes

➤ **PER SERVING** CALORIES: 195; TOTAL FAT: 5G; SATURATED FAT: 1G; TRANS FAT: 0G; CHOLESTEROL: 0MG; SODIUM: 4MG; TOTAL CARBOHYDRATE: 40G; FIBER: 5G; SUGAR: 33G; PROTEIN: 2G

Eating one to two apples per day can lower your LDL (bad) cholesterol levels and raise your HDL (good) levels due to their polyphenols, fiber, and phytosterols. Apples are widely available year-round and are chock full of other healthy nutrients, such as vitamins and minerals, plus they are delicious and make a great snack. This simple recipe dresses up apples with spices and bakes them to enhance their natural sweetness. A healthy alternative to cookies and processed treats, these are especially great in fall and winter when apples are at their peak.

4 large firm, tart apples, such as Winesap, Granny Smith, or Jonagold, halved lengthwise

1 tablespoon freshly squeezed lemon juice

¼ cup pure maple syrup

¼ cup finely chopped, toasted walnuts

1 teaspoon ground cinnamon

½ cup water

1 Preheat the oven to 350°F.

2 With a small knife, remove the core from each apple half, creating a small "basin." Sprinkle the cut sides of the apples with lemon juice and place them in a glass, ceramic, or other nonreactive baking dish.

3 In a small bowl, mix the maple syrup, walnuts, and cinnamon. Fill the apple halves with the nut mixture.

4 Pour the water into the bottom of the baking dish. Cover the apples with aluminum foil or a lid and bake for 25 minutes.

5 Remove the foil and baste the apples with the pan juices. Continue to bake the apples, uncovered, for 10 to 15 minutes more, or until they are tender but not mushy. Let cool slightly before serving.

Substitution tip Vary the spices: Try cloves, ginger, nutmeg, pumpkin pie spice, or a combination of your favorites.

5 MAIN INGREDIENTS	DAIRY FREE	LOW SODIUM

Peanut Butter and Jelly Smoothie

Serves 1 | Prep time: 5 minutes

➤ **PER SERVING** CALORIES: 328; TOTAL FAT: 9G; SATURATED FAT: 2G; TRANS FAT: 0G; CHOLESTEROL: 8MG; SODIUM: 162MG; TOTAL CARBOHYDRATE: 53G; FIBER: 8G; SUGAR: 32G; PROTEIN: 16G

This nutritious, delicious smoothie tastes like a peanut butter and jelly sandwich and takes just minutes to prepare. High in protein, fiber, healthy fats, vitamins, and minerals, the combination of strawberries, Greek yogurt, and peanut butter will satisfy your sandwich craving, but in smoothie form.

1 cup frozen banana slices
   (about 1 medium banana)

½ cup nonfat milk, or plant-based milk

½ cup plain nonfat Greek yogurt

½ cup frozen strawberries

½ cup ice

1 tablespoon natural peanut butter

1 cup fresh baby spinach (optional)

In a high-speed blender, combine the banana, milk, yogurt, strawberries, ice, peanut butter, and spinach (if using). Process until smooth. Enjoy immediately.

Ingredient tip For a sweeter smoothie, add 1 soft, pitted Medjool date or ½ tablespoon pure maple syrup.

30 MINUTES OR FEWER	BUDGET SAVER	LOW SODIUM	ONE POT

Avocado Ice Cream

Serves 2 | Prep time: 5 minutes

➤ **PER SERVING** CALORIES: 247; TOTAL FAT: 14G; SATURATED FAT: 2G; TRANS FAT: 0G; CHOLESTEROL: 0MG; SODIUM: 9MG; TOTAL CARBOHYDRATE: 35G; FIBER: 7G; SUGAR: 21G; PROTEIN: 2G

This creamy, delicious avocado ice cream is made with wholesome ingredients high in cholesterol-lowering fiber, healthy fats, antioxidants, vitamins, and minerals. Naturally sweetened, this is the kind of ice cream you can eat every day and still lower your cholesterol.

1 banana, frozen

1 avocado, peeled, cubed, and frozen

2 tablespoons pure maple syrup

2 tablespoons unsweetened cocoa powder, or cacao powder (optional)

Mint extract, to add (optional)

Coconut flakes, to add (optional)

Nut or seed butter, to add (optional)

1 In a food processor, combine the banana, avocado, maple syrup, and cocoa powder (if using). Process until the ingredients break down and an ice cream consistency is reached. You will need to scrape down the sides during processing.

2 If you are including any add-ins, add them now and continue to process for 2 to 5 minutes more until your desired consistency is reached. Serve.

Did you know? To get the most health benefits from an avocado, peel off the skin, like a banana. This way you get the meat right below the skin.

		5 MAIN INGREDIENTS	30 MINUTES OR FEWER	DAIRY FREE	LOW SODIUM	NUT FREE	

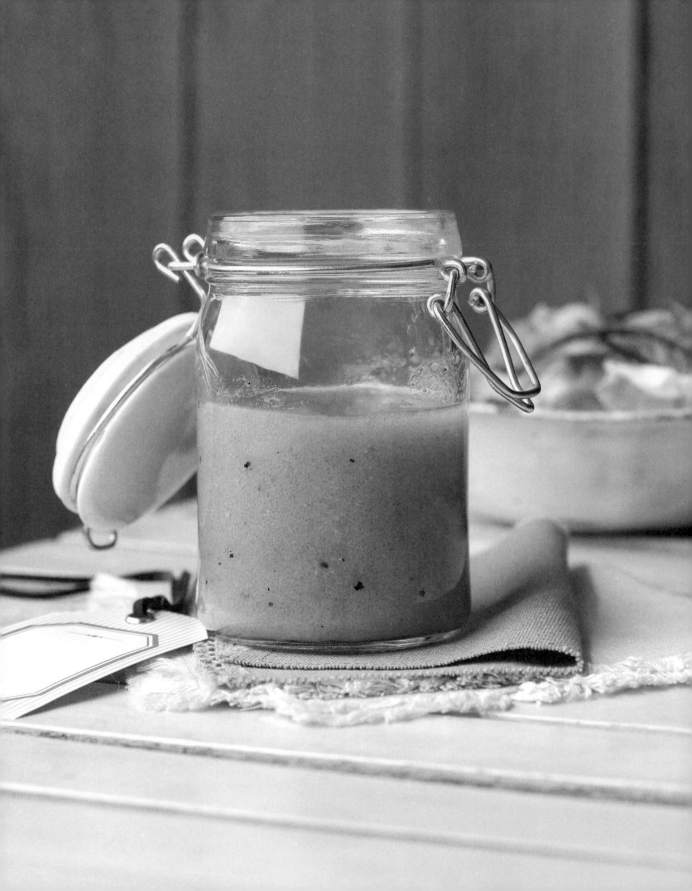

CHAPTER 11

Broths, Condiments, and Sauces

Mustard Vinaigrette

Makes ⅔ cup | Prep time: 30 minutes

➤ **PER SERVING (1 TABLESPOON)** CALORIES: 88; TOTAL FAT: 10G; SATURATED FAT: 2G; TRANS FAT: 0G; CHOLESTEROL: 0MG; SODIUM: 33MG; TOTAL CARBOHYDRATE: 0G; FIBER: 0G; SUGAR: 0G; PROTEIN: 0G

Bottled dressings are typically high in added sugars, fats, sodium, and numerous preservatives, so making your own is a much healthier option. This dressing is simple to assemble and works wonderfully on sturdy greens such as romaine lettuce, or as a topping for cooked vegetables or grains.

1 tablespoon Dijon mustard

2 tablespoons red wine vinegar

1 tablespoon freshly squeezed
   lemon juice

Salt

Freshly ground black pepper

½ cup olive oil

2 garlic cloves, peeled, lightly
   crushed but still intact

2 tarragon sprigs (optional)

1 In a small bowl or measuring cup, combine the Dijon mustard, vinegar, and lemon juice. Season with salt and pepper. Whisk in the olive oil.

2 Add the garlic and tarragon (if using). Marinate for at least 30 minutes. Remove the garlic and tarragon from the dressing before serving.

Ingredient tip If you like your salad dressing a bit sweeter, taste, and adjust to your liking by adding ½ to 1 teaspoon honey. Alternatively, add a pinch or two of sugar.

5 MAIN INGREDIENTS	30 MINUTES OR FEWER	BUDGET SAVER	DAIRY FREE	LOW SODIUM	NUT FREE	ONE POT	

Creamy Avocado Sauce

Makes about 2½ cups | Prep time: 10 minutes

➤ **PER SERVING (¼ CUP)** CALORIES: 110; TOTAL FAT: 11G; SATURATED FAT: 2G; TRANS FAT: 0G; CHOLESTEROL: 0MG; SODIUM: 4MG; TOTAL CARBOHYDRATE: 4G; FIBER: 3G; SUGAR: 0G; PROTEIN: 1G

This creamy avocado sauce is made with just a handful of ingredients and takes less than 10 minutes to prepare. Use as a sauce for zucchini noodles or for whole-grain pasta, grains, or grilled meats and fish. Rich in heart-healthy monounsaturated fats and soluble fiber, this delicious sauce won't have you missing the dairy.

2 avocados, halved, pitted, and peeled

2 garlic cloves, smashed

1 bunch scallions, white and light green parts, roughly chopped

Juice of 1 lemon

¼ cup olive oil

Salt

Freshly ground black pepper

½ cup water

1 In a food processor, combine the avocados, garlic, scallions, lemon juice, and olive oil. Pulse until smooth and season with salt and pepper.

2 Add the water and process until smooth.

3 To serve, place the sauce in a medium pot over low heat and gently warm for 2 to 3 minutes. If using with cooked hot pasta or grains, simply add the sauce to the hot food.

Substitution tip Turn this sauce into a dipping sauce for empanadas or a topping for grilled meat with a Mexican flare by adding 1 bunch of fresh cilantro, 1 teaspoon ground cumin, and 1 to 2 seeded jalapeño or serrano peppers.

5 MAIN INGREDIENTS	30 MINUTES OR FEWER	DAIRY FREE	LOW SODIUM	NUT FREE	ONE POT

Cashew Cream Sauce

Makes 1 cup | Prep time: 10 minutes, plus overnight

➤ **PER SERVING (¼ CUP)** CALORIES: 160; TOTAL FAT: 12G; SATURATED FAT: 2G; TRANS FAT: 0G; CHOLESTEROL: 0MG; SODIUM: 39MG; TOTAL CARBOHYDRATE: 8G; FIBER: 1G; SUGAR: 2G; PROTEIN: 5G

Cashew cream is a healthy cook's secret weapon to creating rich and creamy textures in dishes without the use of full-fat dairy products. You can add cashew cream to just about any sauce or soup to make it extra velvety and smooth, with added garlic for a creamy Alfredo sauce, sweetened and added to smoothies, or used in place of cream cheese. Two flavor combinations are included here (one sweet, one savory), or just blend the cream as is, with no added flavorings.

1 cup raw, unsalted cashews

2½ cups water, divided

⅛ teaspoon salt

OPTIONAL SAVORY FLAVORINGS

2 teaspoons freshly squeezed
    lemon juice

1 garlic clove, minced

Dash paprika

Dash onion powder

OPTIONAL SWEET FLAVORINGS

1 to 2 tablespoons pure maple syrup

1 teaspoon vanilla extract

¼ teaspoon ground cinnamon

1 In a medium bowl, combine the cashews with 2 cups of water. Set aside, uncovered, at room temperature for 10 to 12 hours, or overnight. The cashews are ready when they break apart when pressed between two fingers. Alternately, skip the soak and substitute an equal amount of roasted, unsalted cashews (see tip).

2 Drain the soaking water and transfer the cashews to a blender.

3 Add the savory or sweet flavorings (if using), the remaining ½ cup of water, and the salt. Blend on high speed for about 3 minutes until completely smooth. Stop, scrape down the sides, and process for 1 minute more. Use immediately or transfer to an airtight container and refrigerate for up to 1 week.

Ingredient tip This sauce works great mixed into mashed potatoes, drizzled over scrambled eggs, or as a sandwich spread in place of mayonnaise. You can even freeze cashew cream and turn the cubes into a creamy vegan milkshake. And, to save time, skip the cashew soak (but it does make them easier to digest). Instead, use roasted, unsalted cashews processed with the water in step 3.

5 MAIN INGREDIENTS	DAIRY FREE	LOW SODIUM

Spicy Peanut Sauce

Makes 1⅔ cups | Prep time: 10 minutes

➤ **PER SERVING (¼ CUP)** CALORIES: 199; TOTAL FAT: 14G; SATURATED FAT: 2G; TRANS FAT: 0G; CHOLESTEROL: 0MG; SODIUM: 315MG; TOTAL CARBOHYDRATE: 15G; FIBER: 3G; SUGAR: 9G; PROTEIN: 8G

This spicy peanut sauce is creamy, savory, and completely satisfying, and can serve as the backbone for peanut noodle dishes, as a dip for spring rolls, drizzled on roasted vegetables, used as a delicious dip for veggies, or to top a salad. This does double duty as a sauce or dressing.

¾ cup creamy natural peanut butter

⅓ cup water, plus more as needed

¼ cup rice vinegar

¼ cup low-sodium tamari, or low-sodium soy sauce

3 tablespoons honey, plus more as needed

2 teaspoons grated peeled fresh ginger, or ½ teaspoon ground ginger

2 medium garlic cloves, minced, plus more as needed

¼ teaspoon red pepper flakes

1 In a medium bowl, whisk the peanut butter, water, vinegar, tamari, honey, ginger, garlic, and red pepper flakes until well blended. If your peanut butter is particularly thick, you may need to add a bit more water to thin the mixture. Taste and adjust to your liking with more garlic or honey, as needed. Serve.

Ingredient tip Refrigerate this sauce in an airtight container for up to 1 week. You may need to whisk it again before serving or add a splash of vinegar to perk up the flavors.

	30 MINUTES OR FEWER	BUDGET SAVER	DAIRY FREE	LOW SODIUM	ONE POT	

Easy Tomato-Basil Sauce

Makes 2½ cups | Prep time: 5 minutes | Cook time: 15 minutes

➤ **PER SERVING (½ CUP)**   CALORIES: 73; TOTAL FAT: 6G; SATURATED FAT: 1G; TRANS FAT: 0G; CHOLESTEROL: 0MG; SODIUM: 8MG; TOTAL CARBOHYDRATE: 6G; FIBER: 1G; SUGAR: 1G; PROTEIN: 1G

This quick and easy tomato-basil sauce recipe is designed for busy people with health at the top of their minds. It is entirely possible to have a fresh, healthy meal without spending an hour in the kitchen. You can prepare this extremely versatile recipe as written or add jalapeño peppers (to taste) for a spicy kick. You can use red or white onion and add mushrooms and zucchini for more substance. Full of vitamins, minerals, and fiber, this delicious sauce is perfect on your favorite whole-grain pasta.

2 tablespoons olive oil

½ cup chopped red onion

3 or 4 garlic cloves, minced

2 cups peeled, seeded, chopped
   tomatoes, or canned no-salt-added
   crushed tomatoes

¼ cup fresh basil leaves, chopped

Dash salt

Dash sugar (optional)

1 In a medium saucepan over medium-high heat, heat the olive oil.

2 Add the red onion. Sauté for 2 to 3 minutes, or until it starts to brown.

3 Add the garlic. Sauté for 30 seconds.

4 Carefully add the tomatoes (the juices may cause the hot oil to sputter) and stir to combine. Reduce the heat to low and stir in the basil. Cook for 15 minutes (the sauce should be slightly bubbling).

5 Add the salt and the sugar (if using). Serve with hot pasta.

Ingredient tip To peel tomatoes, bring a pot of water to a boil. With the tip of a sharp paring knife, cut an X into the bottom of each tomato and carefully drop it into the water. Boil for 30 seconds. Remove the tomatoes and quickly run them under cold water. The skins should peel right off.

5 MAIN INGREDIENTS	30 MINUTES OR FEWER	BUDGET SAVER	DAIRY FREE	LOW SODIUM	NUT FREE	ONE POT

Homemade Vegetable Broth

Yield: 8 cups | Prep time: 10 minutes | Cook time: 1 hour

➤ **PER SERVING (1 CUP)** CALORIES: 34; TOTAL FAT: 0G; SATURATED FAT: 0G; TRANS FAT: 0G; CHOLESTEROL: 0MG; SODIUM: 24MG; TOTAL CARBOHYDRATE: 8G; FIBER: 2G; SUGAR: 2G; PROTEIN: 1G

Homemade vegetable broth is a great way to use up vegetable trimmings or potatoes that are about to go bad, cutting down on food waste while providing a healthier alternative to store-bought broth. This basic recipe uses just a handful of ingredients, but you can use other vegetable trimmings you have on hand, including broccoli stalks and kale stems. Use the broth to make soups and gravy, or just to add flavor to your favorite recipes.

2 celery stalks, chopped

1 onion, chopped

1 carrot, chopped

1 medium potato, chopped
    into large chunks

3 or 4 garlic cloves, smashed
    or left whole

8 cups water

Bay leaves, for seasoning (optional)

Peppercorns, for seasoning (optional)

Fresh thyme or fresh parsley,
    for seasoning (optional)

1 In a large pot over high heat, combine the celery, onion, carrot, potato, garlic, water, and seasonings as desired. Bring to a boil. Reduce the heat to low and simmer, covered, for at least 1 hour.

2 Strain out the vegetables and garlic and remove any herbs. Use as needed. Keep refrigerated in an airtight container for up to 1 week.

Ingredient tip Plan ahead: Save your broccoli stems, onion ends, celery bottoms, and potato peels if you know you are going to be making vegetable stock soon. You can also freeze your vegetable odds and ends in a freezer-safe bag or container so they are ready to go when you are, and won't go to waste.

	BUDGET SAVER	DAIRY FREE	LOW SODIUM	NUT FREE	ONE POT	

Mango and Black Bean Salsa

Makes 4 cups | Prep time: 15 minutes

➤ **PER SERVING (¼ CUP)** CALORIES: 34; TOTAL FAT: 0G; SATURATED FAT: 0G; TRANS FAT: 0G;
CHOLESTEROL: 0MG; SODIUM: 1MG; TOTAL CARBOHYDRATE: 7G; FIBER: 2G; SUGAR: 2G; PROTEIN: 2G

Skip the processed salsa and whip up your own flavorful, fiery, fresh version in minutes. Not only are mangos delicious, but they also have high levels of fiber, pectin, and vitamin C, which can lower serum cholesterol levels. Their sweetness balances the spicy flavor of the jalapeño, while black beans add plant protein, fiber, and vitamins and minerals. This salsa is excellent served over homemade burritos or quesadillas, spooned over roasted meat or fish, or enjoyed with tortilla chips.

1 large mango, peeled, pitted, and finely diced

1 (15-ounce) can black beans, drained and rinsed

1 Roma tomato (4 ounces), rinsed, cored, and coarsely chopped

1 fresh jalapeño pepper, seeded and diced

½ cup fresh cilantro, chopped

¼ cup diced red onion

Juice of ½ lime, plus more as needed

Pinch salt, plus more as needed

In a medium bowl, combine the mango, black beans, tomato, jalapeño, cilantro, onion, lime juice, and salt. Gently stir to combine. Cover and refrigerate for at least 10 minutes, and up to 1 day to meld the flavors. Taste the salsa before serving and add more lime juice or salt, if desired.

Substitution tip You can make a number of variations to this recipe depending on your preferences. Try adding 1 peeled, finely diced avocado in place of or in addition to the tomato, add 1 chopped bell pepper, 1 or 2 minced garlic cloves, or even 1 tablespoon red wine vinegar.

	30 MINUTES OR FEWER	BUDGET SAVER	DAIRY FREE	LOW SODIUM	NUT FREE	ONE POT	

Basil Pesto

Makes ½ cup | Prep time: 5 minutes

➤ **PER SERVING (2 TABLESPOONS)** CALORIES: 83; TOTAL FAT: 6G; SATURATED FAT: 1G; TRANS FAT: 0G; CHOLESTEROL: 7MG; SODIUM: 116MG; TOTAL CARBOHYDRATE: 4G; FIBER: 1G; SUGAR: 1G; PROTEIN: 4G

Traditional pesto is quite calorie-dense per serving due to the pine nuts, oil, and cheese used in most recipes. This recipe lightens up the calorie and fat content, while maintaining that distinctive pesto taste and flavor by swapping in nonfat ricotta cheese for some of the Parmesan. If you love pesto, consider making a double batch—it will also be easier to blend that way.

1 cup fresh basil leaves

¼ cup fat-free ricotta cheese

2 tablespoons grated Parmesan cheese

2 tablespoons pine nuts

2 teaspoons olive oil

2 garlic cloves, chopped

⅛ teaspoon salt

¼ teaspoon freshly ground black pepper, plus more as needed

In a blender or food processor, combine the basil, ricotta, Parmesan cheese, pine nuts, olive oil, garlic, salt, and pepper. Process until a smooth paste forms. Refrigerate until ready to serve.

| 30 MINUTES OR FEWER | LOW SODIUM | ONE POT |

Roasted Lemon Sauce

Makes ½ cup | Prep time: 5 minutes | Cook time: 30 minutes

➤ **PER SERVING (¼ CUP)** CALORIES: 221; TOTAL FAT: 22G; SATURATED FAT: 3G; TRANS FAT: 0G; CHOLESTEROL: 0MG; SODIUM: 83MG; TOTAL CARBOHYDRATE: 19G; FIBER: 8G; SUGAR: 11G; PROTEIN: 2G

This creative recipe introduces you to another side of lemons, one you may not be familiar with—their mellow, sweet side brought out through roasting. Made with just three main ingredients, you can use this sauce on almost anything and for just about any type of meal. Drizzle it on grilled foods, use it to top grains, or drizzle it on salads. This recipe makes enough for one or two dinners and will keep in the refrigerator for a few days.

3 medium lemons, halved widthwise, seeds removed

4 garlic cloves, smashed

¼ cup olive oil, divided

⅛ teaspoon salt

1 Arrange a rack in the middle of the oven and preheat the oven to 400°F.

2 Place the lemons cut-side up in a small baking dish. Add the garlic and drizzle with 2 tablespoons of olive oil. Roast for about 30 minutes until the lemons are tender and slightly browned. Remove the baking dish to a wire rack.

3 When the lemons are cool enough to handle, squeeze the juice into the baking dish. Discard the lemon pieces and any remaining seeds. Pour the contents of the baking dish, including the garlic, into a blender or mini food processor.

4 Add the remaining 2 tablespoons of olive oil and salt. Process until the garlic is completely puréed and the sauce is emulsified and slightly thickened. Serve warm or at room temperature.

5 MAIN INGREDIENTS	BUDGET SAVER	DAIRY FREE	LOW SODIUM	NUT FREE

Tahini Sauce

Makes ⅔ cup | Prep time: 5 minutes

➤ **PER SERVING (1 TABLESPOON)** CALORIES: 72; TOTAL FAT: 7G; SATURATED FAT: 1G; TRANS FAT: 0G; CHOLESTEROL: 0MG; SODIUM: 58MG; TOTAL CARBOHYDRATE: 2G; FIBER: 2G; SUGAR: 0G; PROTEIN: 2G

Tahini is a seed butter made from sesame seeds that are hulled, ground, and toasted. It is a major ingredient in hummus, and is extremely versatile for use in many different types of dishes. High in vitamins and minerals, tahini is used in this easy recipe to make a creamy, savory sauce with just three main ingredients. This is the perfect sauce for salads, veggie burgers, roasted vegetables, and grilled meats.

½ cup unsalted tahini

¼ teaspoon salt, plus more
as needed

¼ teaspoon garlic powder,
plus more as needed

1 In a small bowl, whisk the tahini, salt, and garlic powder to combine.

2 Add the water, a little at a time, continuing to whisk, until you have a creamy pourable sauce. Taste and adjust the seasonings as needed. Refrigerate in an airtight container for up to 1 week.

5 MAIN INGREDIENTS	30 MINUTES OR FEWER	BUDGET SAVER	DAIRY FREE	LOW SODIUM	NUT FREE	ONE POT

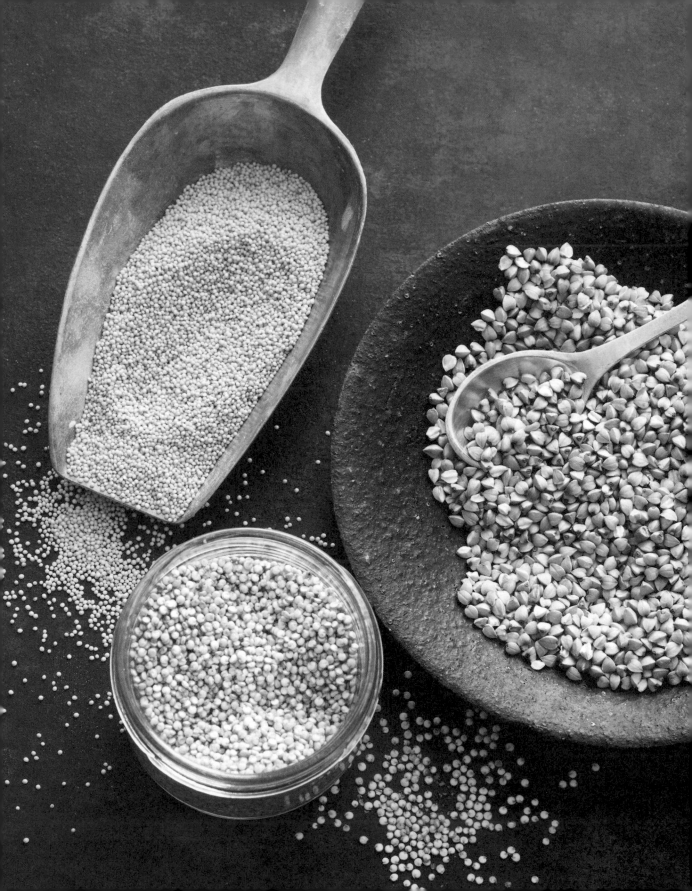

Tips for Dining Out

Whether dining at your family's favorite restaurant or grabbing a snack on the go, you can still make tasty, heart-healthy choices. Following are some dining-out strategies to help. The two big problems to watch for when dining out are saturated fat and salt. Restaurant food is astoundingly high in salt—far more than most people even realize, and many fast-casual restaurant dinners pack upward of 1,500 mg (the daily limit) in one meal! When dining out, it's always important to ask for a low-salt preparation.

How to Order

Scan the menu for low-cholesterol options similar to your at-home preparations—lean proteins, whole grains, lots of fruits and vegetables, and heart-healthy fats. Here are some tips:

- Look for fish or skinless chicken, and choose preparations with little oil. Broiled, baked, grilled, steamed, or poached are healthier than sautéed or fried.

- Order dressings or sauces on the side. To maximize taste, but minimize the amount you eat, dip your fork into the dressing and skewer your salad or food.

- Customize your order. Assume you can have your meal prepared in a different way than listed—you probably can. Ask for your protein grilled instead of fried, for a baked potato instead of fries, or double vegetables instead of fries.

- If you are not sure about the nutritional value of something you're considering, a shortcut is to stay away from dishes with high-fat descriptions such as creamy, *au gratin, au fromage*, breaded, fried, stuffed, or scalloped. And, of course, avoid butter or cheese sauces.

- Drink water or seltzer throughout your meal; it helps you feel fuller faster and helps avoid overeating.

- Bypass high-fat desserts (or just have a bite) in favor of a fruit or sorbet option—or skip it altogether and reward yourself at home with a low-fat indulgence.

Ordering at Your Local Pizza Place or Chinese or Asian Restaurant

Pizza: Order thin crust, ask them to go easy on the cheese, and order vegetable toppings, not meat. So you will feel full without eating too many slices, order a salad—with dressing on the side, of course—and eat it first.

Asian-style foods: Choose main dishes with lots of vegetables and ask for no MSG and no salt. Order healthy proteins such as fish, shrimp, or chicken that are grilled, poached, or steamed (not fried or heavily breaded) with the sauce on the side. Choose vegetable appetizers or dumplings that are steamed, not fried. Avoid any crispy (fried!) noodles often served as an appetizer. Opt for steamed brown rice.

Restaurant Chains and Fast Food

Looking up nutritional data online for your family's favorite restaurant chain or fast food outlet before you go makes it much easier to order heart healthy. No time? No problem—nutritional information is usually available at the restaurant, or on the MyFitnessPal app.

Don't assume menu sections titled "Fit and Healthy" or "Lighter Options" mean lower saturated fat. They may not, and these items are likely laden with salt. To that end, I've researched menu options at some of America's favorite restaurant chains, and included examples of heart-healthier choices later in this section (see page 189).

Snacking on the Run

The best way to quell hunger pangs between meals is with a heart-healthy snack that you've brought from home—Herbed Chickpeas (page 78), or bell pepper strips with a yogurt dip, for example. But if you are out and about, you can still snack smartly. Consider these options:

Grab a piece of fruit. Apples and bananas are available in many places.

Reach for a low-fat yogurt.

Try a hummus and pretzel snack pack.

A SkinnyPop single-serve bag of popcorn delivers 3 grams of dietary fiber.

Choose a heart-healthy snack bar that's made mostly of heart-healthy nuts and seeds and is not laden with sugar.

Stock your handbag, backpack, briefcase, or car with low-fat, high-fiber snacks that travel well:

- Single packs of nuts and seeds (unsalted, of course). If your favorites don't come prepackaged in single servings, make your own using small resealable plastic bags or containers.

- Air pop your own healthy popcorn, and store it in single-serving bags.

- Healthy snack bars made with heart-healthy nuts and seeds and without unhealthy oils. Consider KIND Bars, Luna Bars, LÄRABAR, Clif Bars, Odwalla Bars, some Quaker Bars, Nature Valley Crunchy Granola Bars, and Kashi Bars—but check the nutritional value of your favorite flavor first. Of course, you'll want to ensure bars with chocolate are not left in the hot car or sun!

Wherever you are, these ideas should help make it easier to choose heart-healthy meals and snacks, and stave off hunger between meals.

What to Eat at Your Favorite Restaurant

A bit of online nutritional research before dining out at your family's favorite restaurant chain makes it easier to order heart-healthy foods.

Here are some examples of heart-healthier options at popular American chains: These meal options are low in saturated fat, have no trans fat, and are below the daily sodium recommendation of 1,500 mg.

Following, too, is a list of restaurants with very few heart-healthy menu options, as they are heavily loaded with sodium. (Keep in mind that restaurant menus frequently change.)

Restaurants with Meal Choices Low in Saturated Fat and Below 1,500 mg of Sodium

Bonefish Grill: Just about any of their grilled fish options will be low in saturated fat if you order with either no sauce or the Herb Pesto or Mango Salsa. Snapper with Herb Pesto, for example, has just 3 grams of saturated fat and 500 grams of sodium. Choose Sweet Potato Mash and a steamed green vegetable (ask for no butter or salt added) as sides, and this is a decent low-cholesterol restaurant option.

California Pizza Kitchen: Nearly all pizza has a surprisingly high amount of sodium. That said, half (three slices) of the Wild Mushroom original pizza has 7.5 grams of saturated fat and 1,140 mg of sodium.

Carrabba's Italian Grill: The Tuscan Grilled Chicken with a side of steamed broccoli has just 2 grams of saturated fat and 825 mg of sodium. The Parmesan-Crusted Chicken Arugula has 8 grams of saturated fat and 1,380 mg of sodium.

Chipotle: If you choose low-fat ingredients, there are multiple options at Chipotle. For example, a burrito bowl with no shell, made with chicken, brown rice, black beans, tomatillo-green chile salsa, romaine lettuce, and guacamole has 7.5 grams of saturated fat and 1,340 mg of sodium. To lower the salt and saturated fat, ask for a half serving of guacamole—healthier than cheese or sour cream.

Cracker Barrel: From the "Wholesome Fixin's" section, the Buttermilk Oven-Fried Chicken Breast and Apple Cider BBQ Chicken Breast are healthy choices, with 1 to 2.5 grams of saturated fat and 610 to 630 mg of sodium. Add any steamed vegetable and even their mashed potatoes (no butter or gravy: 2 grams of saturated fat and 170 mg of sodium) for a heart-healthy dinner.

Olive Garden: One of the healthier options on their menu is Herb-Grilled Salmon, with 8 grams of saturated fat and just 570 mg of sodium. There are other chicken, fish, and shrimp options from the "Taste of the Mediterranean" section, most of which are also relatively low in saturated fat but significantly higher in sodium (though all are under 1,500 mg).

Outback Steakhouse: For a surf-and-turf option, their 6-ounce Sirloin and Grilled Shrimp on the Barbie is a decent choice, with 7 grams of saturated fat and 1,010 mg of sodium, if ordered with heart-healthy sides. Better would be the 7-ounce Perfectly Grilled Salmon, with Seasonal Mixed Vegetables, which has 8 grams of saturated fat and 610 mg of sodium.

Red Lobster: The Oven-Broiled Wild-Caught Flounder has just 1 gram of saturated fat and 500 mg of sodium. Similarly, the Shrimp Scampi has 3 grams of saturated fat and 580 mg of sodium.

Ruby Tuesday: All items in their "Fit and Trim" section are very high in sodium. Instead choose the Blackened Tilapia (1 gram of saturated fat and 871 mg sodium) or Grilled Salmon (5 grams of saturated fat and 670 mg sodium) or Hickory Bourbon Chicken or Salmon (4 grams of saturated fat and 432 mg sodium), with steamed vegetables.

Texas Roadhouse: The 6-ounce Choice Sirloin with no Steak Smothers is a decent choice with 2.5 grams of saturated fat and 560 mg of sodium. A sweet potato (no butter) adds 4 grams of saturated fat and 120 mg of sodium. Their Fresh Vegetables pack 7 grams of saturated fat—ask for steamed vegetables, no butter.

TGI Friday's: The Bruschetta Chicken Pasta (7 grams of saturated fat and 840 mg of sodium) is one of their only heart-healthy options. Nearly every other option is either high in saturated fat, high in sodium, or both.

Restaurants with Low-Fat But Very High-Sodium Options

Applebee's: On their "Lighter Fare" menu, the Thai Shrimp Salad has just 3 grams of saturated fat and, although it's their lowest-sodium choice, it still packs 1,670 mg of sodium. Most of their other "Lighter Fare" options are also low in saturated fat, but extremely high in sodium.

Chili's: From their "Lighter Choices" menu, the Margarita Grilled Chicken with steamed broccoli and sweet corn for sides delivers just 2.5 grams of saturated fat, but it has a whopping 3,100 mg of sodium. The only low-fat meal options with less than 1,500 mg of sodium are the Grilled Chicken Salad (6 grams of saturated fat and 1,100 mg of sodium) and the Caribbean Salad with Seared Shrimp or Grilled Chicken (4.5 grams of saturated fat and 1,130 to 1,140 mg of sodium).

The Cheesecake Factory: Their website states, "Where required by law, we provide complete nutritional information in our restaurants. At this time, we do not provide this information on our website." If you can't do the nutritional math, you might not want to eat there.

P. F. Chang's China Bistro: The sodium in nearly every dish is high. The only low-fat dinner options with less than 1,500 mg of sodium are Sweet and Sour Chicken (4.5 grams of saturated fat and 910 mg of sodium) and Crisp Honey Chicken or Korean Chicken Stir-Fry (7 grams of saturated fat and 1,410 mg of sodium).

The Dirty Dozen and Clean Fifteen

A nonprofit environmental watchdog organization called Environmental Working Group (EWG) looks at data supplied by the U.S. Department of Agriculture (USDA) and the Food and Drug Administration (FDA) about pesticide residues. Each year it compiles a list of the best and worst pesticide loads found in commercial crops. You can use these lists to decide which fruits and vegetables to buy organic to minimize your exposure to pesticides and which produce is considered safe enough to buy conventionally. This does not mean they are pesticide-free, though, so wash these fruits and vegetables thoroughly.

DIRTY DOZEN

Apples	Peaches
Celery	Potatoes
Cherry tomatoes	Snap peas (imported)
Cucumbers	Spinach
Grapes	Strawberries
Nectarines (imported)	Sweet bell peppers

In addition to the Dirty Dozen, the EWG added two types of produce contaminated with highly toxic organophosphate insecticides:

Kale/collard greens	Hot peppers

CLEAN FIFTEEN

Asparagus	Kiwis
Avocados	Mangos
Cabbage	Onions
Cantaloupes (domestic)	Papayas
Cauliflower	Pineapples
Eggplants	Sweet corn
Grapefruits	Sweet peas (frozen)
	Sweet potatoes

Measurement Conversions

Volume Equivalents (Liquid)

STANDARD	US STANDARD (OUNCES)	METRIC (APPROXIMATE)
2 tablespoons	1 fl. oz.	30 mL
¼ cup	2 fl. oz.	60 mL
½ cup	4 fl. oz.	120 mL
1 cup	8 fl. oz.	240 mL
1½ cups	12 fl. oz.	355 mL
2 cups or 1 pint	16 fl. oz.	475 mL
4 cups or 1 quart	32 fl. oz.	1 L
1 gallon	128 fl. oz.	4 L

Volume Equivalents (Dry)

STANDARD	METRIC (APPROXIMATE)
⅛ teaspoon	0.5 mL
¼ teaspoon	1 mL
½ teaspoon	2 mL
¾ teaspoon	4 mL
1 teaspoon	5 mL
1 tablespoon	15 mL
¼ cup	59 mL
⅓ cup	79 mL
½ cup	118 mL
⅔ cup	156 mL
¾ cup	177 mL
1 cup	235 mL
2 cups or 1 pint	475 mL
3 cups	700 mL
4 cups or 1 quart	1 L

Oven Temperatures

FAHRENHEIT (F)	CELSIUS (C) (APPROXIMATE)
250°F	120°C
300°F	150°C
325°F	165°C
350°F	180°C
375°F	190°C
400°F	200°C
425°F	220°C
450°F	230°C

Weight Equivalents

STANDARD	METRIC (APPROXIMATE)
½ ounce	15 g
1 ounce	30 g
2 ounces	60 g
4 ounces	115 g
8 ounces	225 g
12 ounces	340 g
16 ounces or 1 pound	455 g

Resources

Cholesterol Basics

The following authorities discuss cholesterol in more detail:

American Heart Association

"About Cholesterol"
www.heart.org/HEARTORG/Conditions
/Cholesterol/AboutCholesterol/About
-Cholesterol_UCM_001220_Article.jsp#
.WbP_29N96i5.

"How Can I Improve My Cholesterol?"
www.heart.org/idc/groups
/heart-public/@wcm/@hcm/documents
/downloadable/ucm_300460.pdf.

**"Prevention and Treatment of High
Cholesterol (Hyperlipidemia)"**
www.heart.org/HEARTORG/Conditions
/Cholesterol/PreventionTreatmentofHigh
Cholesterol/Prevention-and-Treatment
-of-High-Cholesterol-Hyperlipidemia_UCM
_001215_Article.jsp#.WgdJCFtSzIU.

National Heart, Lung, and Blood Institute

"How Is High Blood Cholesterol Diagnosed?"
www.NHLBI.nih.gov/health
/health-topics/topics/hbc/diagnosis.

"What Is Cholesterol?"
www.NHLBI.nih.gov/health/health
-topics/topics/hbc/.

Heart Disease Risk Calculator

Jointly, the American College of Cardiology and the American Heart Association created a calculator for estimating your 10-year risk of atherosclerotic cardiovascular disease (ASCVD). **Important note:** This heart disease calculator is *NOT APPLICABLE* if you take a statin medication and/or have had a heart attack or stroke. To use the calculator, you need to know your:

- Total cholesterol
- LDL cholesterol
- HDL cholesterol
- Systolic blood pressure (the top number)

How to access the ASCVD Risk Calculator:

* On the American Heart Association page at http://static.Heart.org/riskcalc/app/index.html#!/baseline-risk

* Through the Apple and Google Play app stores by searching "ASCVD Risk Estimator Plus"

OR

Available on the American Heart Association page at http://static.Heart.org/riskcalc/app/index.html#!/baseline-risk or through the Apple and Google Play app stores by searching "ASCVD Risk Estimator Plus."

Dietary Guidelines

For overall dietary guidelines, as well as dietary guidelines to specifically lower cholesterol, read more on these websites:

American Heart Association

"The American Heart Association's Diet and Lifestyle Recommendations"
www.heart.org/HEARTORG/HealthyLiving/Diet-and-Lifestyle-Recommendations_UCM_305855_Article.jsp#.WbGR-dN96i5.

The Office of Disease Prevention and Health Promotion

"2015–2020 Dietary Guidelines for Americans."
www.health.gov/dietaryguidelines/2015/.

Eating to Lower Cholesterol

The following websites provide information on how to eat to lower your cholesterol.

American Heart Association

"Cooking to Lower Cholesterol"
www.heart.org/HEARTORG/Conditions/Cholesterol/PreventionTreatmentofHighCholesterol/Cooking-To-Lower-Cholesterol_UCM_305630_Article.jsp.

"Lower Cholesterol with Diet, Foods"
www.GoRedForWomen.org/live-healthy/first-steps-to-prevent-heart-disease-and-be-heart-healthy/lower-cholesterol-with-diet-foods/

Harvard Medical School

"Eleven Foods that Lower Cholesterol"
www.health.harvard.edu/heart-health/11-foods-that-lower-cholesterol.

EatingWell

"Ten Foods that Lower Cholesterol"
www.EatingWell.com/article/288593/10-foods-that-lower-cholesterol/.

Mayo Clinic

"Cholesterol: Top Foods to Improve Your Numbers"
www.MayoClinic.org/diseases-conditions/high-blood-cholesterol/in-depth/cholesterol/art-20045192.

References

Chapter One

High Cholesterol Risk Factors and Target 5 to 6 Percent Saturated Fat Per Day:

American Heart Association. "Prevention and Treatment of High Cholesterol (Hyperlipidemia)." Accessed August 21, 2017. www.heart.org /HEARTORG/Conditions/Cholesterol /PreventionTreatmentofHighCholesterol /Prevention-and-Treatment-of -High-Cholesterol-Hyperlipidemia _UCM_001215_Article.jsp#.WbFOp9N96i5.

Centers for Disease Control and Prevention. "Family History and Other Characteristics That Increase Risk for Heart Disease." Accessed August 21, 2017. www.cdc.gov/heartdisease /family_history.htm.

Centers for Disease Control and Prevention. "High Cholesterol Risk Factors." Accessed August 21, 2017. www.cdc.gov/cholesterol /risk_factors.htm.

National Heart, Lung, and Blood Institute. "Questions and Answers on Cholesterol and Health with NHLBI Nutritionist Janet de Jesus, M.S., R.D." Accessed August 21, 2017. www.nhlbi.nih.gov/news/spotlight/fact-sheet /questions-and-answers-cholesterol-and-health -nhlbi-nutritionist-janet-de-jesus-ms-rd.

Heart Disease Risk Calculator

American Heart Association. "ASCVD Risk Calculator." Accessed August 21, 2017. http://static.heart.org/riskcalc/app/index .html#!/baseline-risk.

Cholesterol Targets

American Heart Association. "Familial Hyper-cholesterolemia (FH)." Accessed August 21, 2017. www.heart.org/HEARTORG/Conditions /Cholesterol/CausesofHighCholesterol /Familial-Hypercholesterolemia-FH _UCM_493541_Article.jsp.

Mayo Clinic. "Triglycerides: Why Do They Matter?" Accessed October 1, 2017. www .mayoclinic.org/diseases-conditions /high-blood-cholesterol/in-depth /triglycerides/art-20048186.

National Heart, Lung, and Blood Institute. "High Blood Cholesterol: What You Need to Know." Accessed August 21, 2017. www.nhlbi.nih.gov /health/resources/heart/heart-cholesterol -hbc-what-html.

Cholesterol Medication

Mayo Clinic. "Cholesterol Medications: Consider the Options." Accessed August 21, 2017. www.mayoclinic.org/diseases-conditions /high-blood-cholesterol/in-depth /cholesterol-medications/art-20050958.

Fats: Saturated and Trans Fats

American Heart Association. "The Skinny on Fats." Accessed August 21, 2017. www.heart.org /HEARTORG/Conditions/Cholesterol /PreventionTreatmentofHighCholesterol /The-Skinny-on-Fats_UCM_305628_Article .jsp#.WbFZ09N96i4.

High Cholesterol versus Dietary Cholesterol

National Heart, Lung, and Blood Institute. "Questions and Answers on Cholesterol and Health with NHLBI Nutritionist Janet de Jesus, M.S., R.D." Accessed August 21, 2017. www.nhlbi.nih.gov/news/spotlight/fact-sheet /questions-and-answers-cholesterol-and-health -nhlbi-nutritionist-janet-de-jesus-ms-rd.

Trans Fats No Longer GRAS

US Food and Drug Administration. "FDA Cuts Trans Fat in Processed Foods." Accessed August 21, 2017. www.fda.gov/ForConsumers /ConsumerUpdates/ucm372915.htm.

Foods That Lower Cholesterol (and No Trans Fats)

Harvard Health Publications, Harvard Medical School. "Eleven Foods That Lower Cholesterol." Accessed August 21, 2017. www.health.harvard .edu/heart-health/11-foods-that-lower -cholesterol.

Margolis, Lindsay. "Ten Foods that Lower Cholesterol." EatingWell. Accessed August 29, 2017. www.eatingwell.com/article /288593/10-foods-that-lower-cholesterol/.

Sugar and Salt Intake

American Heart Association. "Added Sugars Add to Your Risk of Dying from Heart Disease." Accessed August 21, 2017. www.heart.org /HEARTORG/HealthyLiving/HealthyEating /Nutrition/Added-Sugars-Add-to-Your-Risk -of-Dying-from-Heart-Disease_UCM_460319 _Article.jsp#.WbFfU9N96i6.

American Heart Association. "Sodium and Salt." Accessed August 21, 2017. www.heart.org /HEARTORG/HealthyLiving/HealthyEating /Nutrition/Sodium-and-Salt_UCM_303290 _Article.jsp.

Centers for Disease Control and Prevention. "Get the Facts: Sodium's Role in Processed Food." Accessed September 9, 2017. www.cdc.gov/salt /pdfs/sodium_role_processed.pdf.

Mayo Clinic Recommends 1,500 mg Salt for Lower-Sodium DASH Diet

(Note: This DASH diet also has the recommended servings per day of each food element.)

Mayo Clinic. "DASH Diet: Healthy Eating to Lower Your Blood Pressure." Accessed August 27, 2017. www.mayoclinic.org/healthy-lifestyle /nutrition-and-healthy-eating/in-depth /dash-diet/art-20048456.

American Heart Association Salt Recommendation: 1,500 mg of Salt

American Heart Association. "Why Should I Limit Sodium?" Accessed August 27, 2017. www.heart.org/idc/groups/heart-public /@wcm/@hcm/documents/downloadable /ucm_300625.pdf.

What to Eat to Lower Cholesterol

American Heart Association. "Cooking to Lower Cholesterol." Accessed August 21, 2017. www.heart.org/HEARTORG/Conditions /Cholesterol/PreventionTreatmentofHigh Cholesterol/Cooking-To-Lower-Cholesterol _UCM_305630_Article.jsp.

American Heart Association Go Red for Women. "Lower Cholesterol with Diet, Foods." Accessed August 21, 2017. www.goredforwomen.org /live-healthy/first-steps-to-prevent-heart -disease-and-be-heart-healthy/lower -cholesterol-with-diet-foods/.

Dr. Oz. "Top 10 Food to Lower Cholesterol." Accessed August 21, 2017. http://www.doctoroz .com/slideshow/top-10-foods-lower-cholesterol.

Mayo Clinic. "Cholesterol: Top Foods to Improve Your Numbers." Accessed August 21, 2017. www.mayoclinic.org/diseases-conditions /high-blood-cholesterol/in-depth/cholesterol /art-20045192. (Note: contains fiber information: 5 to 10 grams/day reduces LDL cholesterol).

Office of Disease Prevention and Health Promotion. "2015–2020 Dietary Guidelines for Americans." Accessed August 27, 2017. www.health.gov/dietaryguidelines/2015/

American Heart Association on Diet to Lower Blood Cholesterol (5 to 6 Percent Saturated Fat = 13g)

American Heart Association. "The American Heart Association's Diet and Lifestyle Recom- mendations." Accessed August 21, 2017. www.heart.org/HEARTORG/HealthyLiving /Diet-and-Lifestyle-Recommendations _UCM_305855_Article.jsp#.WbGR-dN96i5.

Heart Disease Risk Factors (and for Women, Menopause Risk Increase)

National Heart, Lung, and Blood Institute. "What Are the Risk Factors for Heart Disease? Accessed August 31, 2017. www.nhlbi.nih.gov /health/educational/hearttruth/lower-risk /risk-factors.htm.

Fiber

SOLUBLE VERSUS INSOLUBLE FIBER

Gardner, Amanda. "Soluble and Insoluble Fiber: What's the Difference?" WebMD. Accessed August 30, 2017. www.webmd.com/diet /features/insoluble-soluble-fiber.

HOW MUCH FIBER (OLDER PEOPLE NEED LESS)

Mayo Clinic. "Dietary Fiber: Essential for a Healthy Diet." Accessed August 30, 2017. www.mayoclinic.org/healthy-lifestyle /nutrition-and-healthy-eating/in-depth/fiber /art-20043983?pg=1.

US Department of Agriculture. "2015–2020 Dietary Guidelines for Americans." Accessed August 27, 2017. https://health.gov /dietaryguidelines/2015.

American Heart Association. "Whole Grains and Fiber." Accessed September 6, 2017. www.heart .org/HEARTORG/HealthyLiving/Healthy Eating/HealthyDietGoals/Whole-Grains -and-Fiber_UCM_303249_Article.jsp# .Wa57eNOGOi5.

Dahl, W. J., and M. L. Stewart. "Position of the Academy of Nutrition and Dietetics: Health Implications of Dietary Fiber." Accessed August 27, 2017. Journal of the Academy of Nutrition and Dietetics 115, no. 11 (November 2015): 1861–70. doi:10.1016/j.jand.2015.09.003.

Sidebar: Cholesterol

National Heart, Lung, and Blood Institute. "How Is High Blood Cholesterol Diagnosed?" Accessed August 29, 2017. www.nhlbi.nih.gov/health /health-topics/topics/hbc/diagnosis.

Cholesterol-Lowering Medications

American Heart Association. "Cholesterol Medications." Accessed August 29, 2017. www.heart.org/HEARTORG/Conditions /Cholesterol/PreventionTreatmentofHigh Cholesterol/Cholesterol-Medications _UCM_305632_Article.jsp#.WaWrM5OGOi4.

Mayo Clinic. "Cholesterol Medications: Consider the Options." Accessed August 29, 2017. www.mayoclinic.org/diseases-conditions /high-blood-cholesterol/in-depth /cholesterol-medications/art-20050958.

Amount of Saturated Fat per Day

National Heart, Lung, and Blood Institute. "Your Guide to Lowering Your Cholesterol with Therapeutic Lifestyle Changes (TLC)." Accessed September 3, 2017. www.nhlbi.nih.gov/health /resources/heart/cholesterol-tlc.

Fast Food

Wendy's nutritional information: Menu.wendys. com. Accessed August 31, 2017.

- menu.wendys.com/en_US/product /daves-single/

- menu.wendys.com/en_US/product /grilled-chicken-sandwich/

- menu.wendys.com/en_US/product /french-fries/

- menu.wendys.com/en_US/product /chocolate-frosty/

McDonald's nutritional information: www
.mcdonalds.com/us/en-us.html. Accessed
August 31, 2017.

Chapter Two

Heart-Checkmark Program

American Heart Association. "Heart-Check Food
Certification Program Nutrition Requirements."
Accessed September 1, 2107. www.heart.org
/HEARTORG/HealthyLiving/HealthyEating
/Heart-CheckMarkCertification/Heart-Check
-Food-Certification-Program-Nutrition
-Requirements_UCM_300914_Article.jsp.

American Heart Association. "How the
Heart-Check Food Certification Program Works."
Accessed September 1, 2017. www.heart.org
/HEARTORG/HealthyLiving/HealthyEating
/Heart-CheckMarkCertification/How-the
-Heart-Check-Food-Certification-Program
-Works_UCM_300133_Article.jsp.

Low-Fat Food Designation

US Food and Drug Administration. "Guidance
for Industry: A Food Labeling Guide." Accessed
September 4, 2017. www.fda.gov/Food
/GuidanceRegulation/GuidanceDocuments
RegulatoryInformation/LabelingNutrition
/ucm064911.htm.

Pantry Cleanup

American Heart Association. "Expert Tips
for Following Your 2017 Healthy-Eating
Resolutions." Accessed September 1, 2017.

https://news.heart.org/expert-tips-for-following
-your-2017-healthy-eating-resolutions/

Peanut Butter

Eat This, Not That. "The 36 Top Peanut Butters—
Ranked!" Accessed September 3, 2017.
www.eatthis.com/peanut-butter-ranked.

Trader Joe's. "Organic Creamy Salted Peanut
Butter." Accessed September 3, 2017.
www.traderjoes.com/fearless-flyer/article/2152.

Nut Butters: Less Saturated Fat than Peanut Butter

Vegetarian Times. "Nut Butters 101." Accessed
September 23, 2017. www.vegetariantimes.com
/skills/food-fight-almond-vs-peanut-vs
-cashew-butter.

Butter versus Margarine

Cleveland Clinic. "Margarine or Butter: The
Heart-Healthiest Spreads." Accessed September
5, 2017. https://health.clevelandclinic.org
/2014/01/margarine-or-butter-the-heart
-healthiest-spreads-infographic/.

Eggs

Amidor, Toby. "Egg Yolks: To Eat or Toss?" *US
News & World Report*. Accessed September 5,
2017. https://health.usnews.com/health-news
/blogs/eat-run/2014/05/30/egg-yolks-to
-eat-or-toss.

US National Library of Medicine National Institutes of Health. "Egg Consumption and Heart Health: A Review." Accessed September 5, 2017. www.ncbi.nlm.nih.gov/pubmed/28359368.

Exercise

American Heart Association. "American Heart Association Recommendations for Physical Activity in Adults." Accessed September 6, 2017. www.heart.org/HEARTORG/HealthyLiving /PhysicalActivity/FitnessBasics/American -Heart-Association-Recommendations-for -Physical-Activity-in-Adults_UCM_307976 _Article.jsp#.WbAT4dOGOi4.

American Heart Association. "Moderate to Vigorous—What Is Your Level of Intensity?" Accessed September 6, 2017. www.heart.org /HEARTORG/HealthyLiving/PhysicalActivity /FitnessBasics/Moderate-to-Vigorous---What -is-your-level-of-intensity_UCM_463775 _Article.jsp#.WbATodOGOi4.

American Heart Association. "Strength and Resistance Training Exercise." Accessed September 6, 2017. www.heart.org/HEARTORG /HealthyLiving/PhysicalActivity/Fitness Basics/Strength-and-Resistance-Training -Exercise_UCM_462357_Article.jsp# .WbA3Z9N95EI.

Centers for Disease Control and Prevention. "General Physical Activities Defined by Level of Intensity." Accessed September 6, 2017. www.cdc.gov/nccdphp/dnpa/physical/pdf /pa_intensity_table_2_1.pdf.

Stretching

Mayo Clinic: "Hamstring Stretch." Accessed October 6, 2017. www.mayoclinic.org /hamstring-stretch/img-20006930.

Mayo Clinic. "Slideshow: A Guide to Basic Stretches." Accessed September 6, 2017. www .mayoclinic.org/healthy-lifestyle/fitness /multimedia/stretching/sls-20076840.

Appendix A

Aubrey, Allison. "Why the FDA Is Re-Evaluating the Nutty Definition of Healthy Food." National Public Radio. Accessed to October 6, 2017. www .npr.org/sections/thesalt/2016/05/10 /477514200/why-the-fda-is-reevaluating -the-nutty-definition-of-healthy-food.

Food Network. "Healthier Options at Chain Restaurants." Accessed September 12, 2017. www.foodnetwork.com/restaurants/photos /healthy-restaurant-menus.

Narins, Elizabeth. "Fifteen Healthy Restaurant Meals that Aren't Salad." *Cosmopolitan*. August 28, 2015. Accessed September 12, 2017. www .cosmopolitan.com/health-fitness/a45480 /healthy-meals-that-arent-salad/.

Reader's Digest. "20 Tricks to Eating Healthy While Eating Out." Accessed September 12, 2017. www.rd.com/health/healthy-eating/eating -out-healthy/.

Snacking

Eat This, Not That. "Every Kind of Bar Ranked." Accessed September 15, 2017. www.eatthis.com /kind-bars.

Kelly, Diana. "Seven Low-Sugar Granola Bars to Stock Up on for Healthy Snacking." Prevention. com. May 11, 2017. Accessed September 15, 2017. www.prevention.com/food/low-sugar -granola-bars.

SkinnyPop. Accessed September 15, 2017. www .skinnypop.com/foodservice/single-serve-bag/.

Tucker, Alexa. "The FDA Says KIND Bars are Healthy Again." Self.com. May 11, 2016. Accessed October 6, 2017. www.self.com/story/the-fda -says-kind-bars-are-healthy-again.

Restaurant Chains: Nutritional Info

Applebee's: www.applebees.com /nutritional-info.

Bonefish Grill: http://bonefishgrill.blob.core .windows.net/menu/bonefishgrill_nutritional _information.pdf.

California Pizza Kitchen: www.cpk.com /Contents/Downloads/Nutrition-Allergen.pdf.

Carrabba's Italian Grill: www.carrabbas.com /menu/nutrition/ and carrabbas.blob.core. windows.net/assets/menus/May_nutrition _information_for_website_adjusted_082017.pdf.

Chili's: www.chilis.com/docs/Chilis -Nutrition-Menu-Generic.pdf.

Chipotle: www.chipotle.com/nutrition-calculator.

Cracker Barrel: www.crackerbarrel.com /search?searchText=nutrition.

Olive Garden: www.media.olivegarden.com /en_us/pdf/olive_garden_nutrition.pdf.

Outback Steakhouse: https://outback.blob.core .windows.net/content/images/OBS_Full _Nutrition_Information_Core_Menu_Items.pdf.

P. F. Chang's China Bistro: www.pfchangs.com /menu/nutrition/main-menu/.

The Cheesecake Factory: https://www.the cheesecakefactory.com/connect/got-questions/.

Red Lobster: www.redlobster.com /nutrition-tools/interactive-menu.

Ruby Tuesday: www.gipsee.com/rubytnutrition /MenuCategoryGroup.aspx?uid=&loc =LOCATION+%7c+811+Bridgeport+Ave.%2c +Shelton%2c+CT+06484&sid=3777.

Texas Roadhouse: www.texasroadhouse.com /docs/default-source/default-document- library/txrh-nutritional-guide.pdf.

TGI Friday's: www.tgifridays.com/pdf /nutrition.pdf.

Recipe Index

Index

About the Authors

In 2010, **KAREN SWANSON** was stunned by her doctor's recommendation that she consider statin medication due to a sudden spike in her cholesterol levels. Believing (well, at that point, hoping) that, despite her family history, she could naturally lower cholesterol with lifestyle changes, Karen began to research and write about cholesterol.

She has since written articles for Healthline and served as Category Expert for Answers.com. Her award-winning blog, GoLowCholesterol.com, explores cholesterol issues in plain terms and shares tips for lowering cholesterol through what she calls a "lo-co" food and exercise lifestyle. An avid home cook, Karen is always on the hunt for low-fat, easy, delicious recipes.

As for her own lo-co experience, Karen has successfully staved off statin medication with near-daily exercise, learning to love (okay, tolerate) a daily fiber supplement, replacing half-and-half with soy creamer, mostly ditching red meat, and relinquishing her beloved Phish Food ice cream. But she still enjoys wine and chocolate—in moderation, of course.

JENNIFER KOSLO is a Registered Dietitian Nutritionist (RDN), Board Certified Specialist in Sports Dietetics (CSSD), Licensed Dietitian in the state of Texas, and an American Council on Exercise Certified Personal Trainer. A member of the Sports, Cardiovascular, and Wellness Practice Group of the Academy of Nutrition and Dietetics (SCAN), she holds a Doctorate of Philosophy in education and a dual Master of Science degree in Exercise Science and Human Nutrition.

Jennifer's experience includes almost three years as a US Peace Corps fisheries volunteer in Sierra Leone, West Africa; as a cardiac dietitian in clinical nutrition; as the chronic disease nutritionist for a state health department; as a college professor teaching nutrition and sports nutrition; and as a private-practice dietitian doing one-on-one nutrition counseling.

Author of eight healthy eating cookbooks: *The 21-Day Healthy Smoothie Plan*, *The Diabetic Cooking for Two*, *The Healthy Smoothie Recipe Book*, *The Alkaline Diet for Beginners*, *The Insulin Resistance Diet for PCOS*, *The Heart Healthy Cookbook for Two*, *The DASH Diet for Beginners*, and *Lower Your Blood Pressure*, Jennifer continues to teach college-level nutrition and sports nutrition, writes, and provides individual nutrition counseling and personal training services through her online business, Koslo's Nutrition Solutions.